Recent Advances in

Endocrinology and Diabetes 1

Recent Advances in

Endocrinology and Diabetes 1

Amir H Sam MRCP PhD SFHEA
Consultant Endocrinologist
Division of Diabetes, Endocrinology and Metabolism
Hammersmith Hospital, London, UK
Reader in Endocrinology
Imperial College London, London, UK

Saira Hameed MA (Oxon) MRCP PhD FHEA
NIHR Clinical Lecturer
Division of Diabetes, Endocrinology and Metabolism
Imperial College London, London, UK

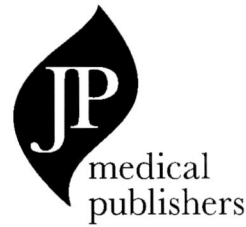

JP
medical
publishers

London • Panama City • New Delhi

© 2017 JP Medical Ltd.
Published by JP Medical Ltd,
83 Victoria Street, London, SW1H 0HW, UK
Tel: +44 (0)20 3170 8910
Fax: +44 (0)20 3008 6180
Email: info@jpmedpub.com
Web: www.jpmedpub.com

ISBN: 978-1-909836-52-5

British Library Cataloguing in Publication Data
A catalogue record for this book is available from the British Library

Library of Congress Cataloging in Publication Data
A catalog record for this book is available from the Library of Congress

Commissioning Editor:	Steffan Clements
Editorial Assistant:	Adam Rajah
Design:	Designers Collective Ltd

Preface

Endocrinology continues to be a highly dynamic and evolving specialty. The revolutions in molecular biology and genomics have given new insights into the physiology and pathophysiology of the endocrine system as well as providing a framework for rational drug development. One of the challenges and excitements of the discipline is that endocrinology is not limited to a specific organ but rather showcases the response of many systems to hormonal turmoil. Furthermore, the idiosyncratic nature of the body's response to hormone deficiency or excess means that no two cases are ever the same.

In this volume, we have distilled hundreds of publications as well as clinical experience into ten chapters encompassing areas within endocrinology which are moving apace. We hope that in this age of information excess, the wisdom of the authors contextualises the wealth of new and ever-emerging knowledge within a practical evidence-based narrative.

Our collective intention has been to appeal to specialists but also to share with non-specialists and medical students the exciting progress in the field. We hope as you read about these recent advances that you not only discover the known knowns but ponder the known unknowns which may yet reveal their secrets with each year of human endeavour.

Amir H Sam
Saira Hameed
January 2017

Contents

Chapter 1

Familial pituitary tumours

Victoria Salem, Harvinder Chahal

INTRODUCTION

Pituitary tumours are common intracranial neoplasms and constitute an important case load in any endocrine clinic. Meta-analysis of autopsy and radiological studies suggest their occurrence is 14–22% in adults. A small but significant proportion of these will manifest clinically, with an estimated prevalence of 1 in 1000 of the population. Although usually histologically benign, these adenomas have a significant burden in terms of disease effects (hormonal excess/deficiency and mass effects) and treatment (neurosurgery, lifelong drug requirements and radiotherapy). Furthermore, there is increasing recognition that some pituitary tumours may occur in a familial setting, possibly as part of a more widespread endocrine neoplastic syndrome [1]. In this chapter, we will focus on those estimated 5% of pituitary adenomas that are familial in origin. We will begin with a brief reminder of pituitary tumour classification before moving on to highlight recent advances in our understanding of genetic syndromes which predispose to pituitary adenomas.

PITUITARY TUMOUR CLASSIFICATION SYSTEMS

Anterior pituitary tumours are usually classified clinically by their hormone secreting type. The most common is the prolactinoma (40–50%). A further one-third is not associated with any hypersecretion of hormones [nonfunctioning pituitary ademonas (NFPAs)]. Growth hormone (GH) secreting or adrenocorticotropic hormone (ACTH)-secreting adenomas account for 10–15% of all pituitary adenomas while thyrotropin-secreting pituitary tumours (TSH-omas) are very rare. These tumours may also be classified according to their size (microadenomas are < 10 mm versus macroadenomas, which are > 10 mm).

The 2004 World Health Organization classification of pituitary tumours requires the identification of transcription factors that regulate cell differentiation and hormone production [2]. These are the oestrogen receptor (ER), thyrotroph embryonic factor (TEF), steroidogenic factor (SF), pituitary-specific positive transcription factor 1 (Pit-1) and pituitary-restricted transcription factor (T-pit). This allows for the classification of pituitary tumours in terms of their cytodifferentiation and also allows for the fairly common phenomenon of plurihormonal adenoma. However, although a number of genetic

Victoria Salem PhD MEd MRCP, Division of Diabetes, Endocrinology and Metabolism, Imperial College London, UK.

Harvinder Chahal PhD MRCP, Division of Diabetes, Endocrinology and Metabolism, Imperial College London, UK. Email: harvinder. chahal@imperial.nhs.uk (for correspondence).

mutations or the abnormal expression of cellular regulators have been implicated in the aetiology of sporadic pituitary adenomas, none have been definitively shown to confer a unique or vital involvement in the primary pathogenetic process.

By contrast, the past 15 years have witnessed many advances in our understanding of familial pituitary adenoma syndromes and their associated gene mutations (summarised in **Figure 1.1**). This is important for the advancement of our global understanding of normal pituitary physiology as well as the pathophysiology of pituitary adenomas occurring outside these specific genetic settings (i.e. sporadic pituitary adenomas). Endocrinologists should be aware that pituitary tumours that occur in this context may display more aggressive behaviour and reduced response to therapy. Clinicians must also understand the requirements for clinical screening for potential associated pathologies and genetic screening in both the index case and their first-degree relatives.

MULTIPLE ENDOCRINE NEOPLASIA TYPE-1

Multiple endocrine neoplasia type 1 (MEN-1) is an autosomal dominant syndrome that is caused by an inactivating mutation in the MEN-1 gene located on chromosome 11q13. The main components are parathyroid (most common), pancreatic and pituitary tumours, and a typically high penetrance, with over 95% of patients manifesting clinically by the age of 50 years. A clinical diagnosis requires the presence of at least two of the component tumours

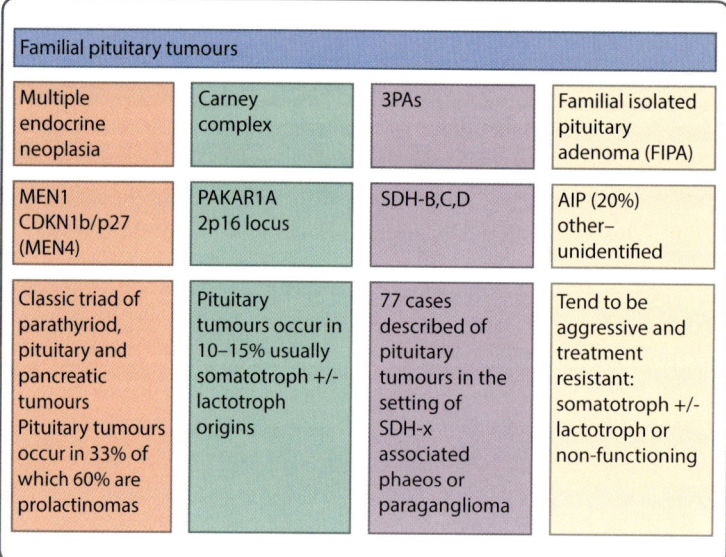

Familial pituitary tumours			
Multiple endocrine neoplasia	Carney complex	3PAs	Familial isolated pituitary adenoma (FIPA)
MEN1 CDKN1b/p27 (MEN4)	PAKAR1A 2p16 locus	SDH-B,C,D	AIP (20%) other– unidentified
Classic triad of parathyriod, pituitary and pancreatic tumours Pituitary tumours occur in 33% of which 60% are prolactinomas	Pituitary tumours occur in 10–15% usually somatotroph +/- lactotroph origins	77 cases described of pituitary tumours in the setting of SDH-x associated phaeos or paraganglioma	Tend to be aggressive and treatment resistant: somatotroph +/- lactotroph or non-functioning

Figure 1.1 Summary of familial pituitary tumour syndromes, identified mutations and classic clinical presentation. Approximately 5% of all pituitary tumours occur in a familial setting and are the result of a germline genetic mutation often arising in tumor suppressor genes. Mutations in the MEN-1 gene or rarely in the CDKN1B (coding for cell cycle regulator protein p27) gene cause MEN-1 and MEN-4 respectively, although in a small proportion of affected cases, no gene abnormality can be found. Carney complex is associated with a mutation in the protein kinase A regulatory subunit gene (PRKAR1A) in 60% affected patients. Linkage studies have suggested a causative gene in the 2q16 area of the remaining 40%. Patients have also been described with familial pituitary adenomas in the setting of classical SDH mutation-related familial paraganglioma/phaeochromocytoma. Families with pituitary tumours that do not fit into the above categories have been grouped together under the diagnosis of familial isolated pituitary adenomas (FIPA). 20% of these families have a mutation in the aryl-hydrocarbon receptor-interacting protein (AIP) gene; in the remaining families the causative gene has not yet been identified.

and a first-degree relative with one of those tumours, although modern genetic testing may now pre-empt this. Pituitary adenomas occur in around a third of MEN-1 patients, with prolactinomas being the most common (60%), followed by somatotroph adenomas (20%), while < 15% are corticotroph or nonfunctioning pituitary adenomas. Conversely, fewer than 3% of all patients diagnosed with sporadic anterior pituitary tumours will have MEN-1 (such that MEN-1 screening is not recommended in these cases). MEN-1 affects both sexes equally but the pituitary manifestation, most commonly prolactinomas, has a female preponderance and sometimes paediatric onset (as early as 5 years of age). Pituitary adenomas are the first presentation of MEN-1 syndrome in about 14% of cases [3].

The pituitary tumours associated with MEN-1 are commonly reported to present younger, and to be larger, plurihormonal, more aggressive and less responsive to therapy than sporadic pituitary tumours [4], although there is no evidence that they are more likely to be malignant. However, a recent large Dutch cohort study in 2015 of 323 people with MEN-1 found the prevalence of pituitary tumours to be 38%, with approximately two thirds of them being microadenomas. These patients were being looked after in modern multi-disciplinary endocrine clinics, and many will have been diagnosed through a screening programme. In such a setting, the pituitary tumours detected were predominantly nonfunctioning microadenomas that did not require treatment [5].

The MEN-1 gene was first identified in 1997 [6]. It is a tumour-suppressor gene, therefore, a somatic mutation to the second allele of MEN-1 in addition to the germline MEN-1 mutation is required for tumourigenesis to occur. The function of its gene product, menin, is still poorly understood. Multiple roles have been proposed, including regulation of gene transcription, cell proliferation, apoptosis and genome stability. The effects of menin on the regulation of the cyclin-dependent kinase inhibitors p27 and p18 may be particularly relevant, given that loss of these in mouse models results in a MEN-1 like syndrome [7]. However, the disparity between the ubiquitous expression of this nuclear protein and the restricted pattern of endocrine tumours in MEN-1 syndrome remains unexplained.

Over 1300 mutations in the MEN-1 gene have been identified throughout the entire coding region and splice sites, with many newly identified mutations in 2015 [8-12]. The majority of MEN-1 mutations are likely to produce a truncated and dysfunctional form of menin, which is unable to interact normally with other proteins by which it alters critical events in cell cycle regulation and proliferation. The chances of detecting a *MEN-1* mutation in an individual is predicted by their clinical presentation, ranging from 3% in people with an apparent sporadic pituitary adenoma to 69% if all three component MEN-1 tumours are present (parathyroid, pancreatic and pituitary) to > 90% in patients with the three component tumours and a positive family history. The most common mutation is a four base-pair deletion (c.249–252 delGTCT) that occurs in 4.5% of patients with MEN1 [13]. Initial comparisons of clinical features in patients and family members with the same MEN-1 mutations have not revealed any genotype–phenotype correlations. However, a recent study of 797 MEN-1 patients from 265 kindred found significant intrafamilial correlations for pituitary adenomas and 65% heritability, suggesting the existence of as-yet-unidentified modifying genetic factors for pituitary MEN-1 tumour types [14].

Current guidance suggests that all MEN-1 mutation carriers should be considered at high risk of developing pituitary tumours. Recommended screening is with annual biochemical monitoring of serum prolactin and IGF-1, and MRI of the pituitary every 3 years [4]. Since the earliest manifestation of MEN-1 related tumours has been reported in children as young as 5 years old, genetic testing of first-degree relatives is recommended as soon as possible.

MULTIPLE ENDOCRINE NEOPLASIA TYPE-4

Multiple endocrine neoplasia type 4 (MEN-4) is an extremely rare familial syndrome seen in patients with MEN1-like features, but no MEN-1 gene mutations. A few such cases have been identified as resulting from mutations in genes coding for cyclin-dependent kinase inhibitors (CDKIs), such as p15, p18, and p21 and p27 [15,16]. The molecular mechanisms by which these cell cycle regulators contribute to endocrine tumourigenesis remains unclear, although *CDKN1B*/p27 is known to interact with the menin protein which may explain the similar phenotype to MEN-1. More recently, 2 out of 124 patients with aryl-hydrocarbon receptor-interacting protein (AIP) mutation negative familial isolated pituitary adenoma (FIPA) (see *Familial isolated pituitary adenomas* section) were screened and found to have cyclin-dependent kinase inhibitor 1B (*CDKN1B*) mutations [17]. However, the low incidence and lack of clear prognostic implications of this mutation makes it unlikely to be of use in routine genetic investigation of familial pituitary tumour syndromes [18].

CARNEY COMPLEX

Carney complex (CNC) is a rare multiple neoplasia syndrome, occurring sporadically (in 30% of cases) or otherwise inherited in an autosomal-dominant manner with 100% penetrance. There are approximately 750 cases described worldwide [19]. CNC is characterised by pigmented lesions of the skin and mucosae, myxomatous tumors (particularly of the cardiac atria), and multiple endocrine neoplasms, including pituitary tumours. Up to 75% of patients with CNC have mildly elevated circulating levels of GH, IGF-1 or prolactin without radiological evidence of a pituitary tumour. Acromegaly ultimately develops in 10–12% of these patients, usually after the third decade of life, and the pituitary tumours in CNC patients operated on for acromegaly confirm somatolactotrophic hyperplasia as the preceding pathology.

More than 70% of patients diagnosed with CNC carry a mutation in the tumour suppressor *PRKAR1A* gene on chromosome 17, which codes for the regulatory subunit type Iα of the cAMP-dependent protein kinase A (PKA) enzyme. Its precise role in the development of CNC is unclear. To date, more than 125 pathogenic *PRKAR1A* mutations have been reported, most of which are unique (i.e. presenting in a single family) [20,21]. Linkage analysis in *PRKAR1A*-negative patients with CNC has revealed another locus at chromosome 2p16 [22], although the gene residing in that part of the chromosome responsible for the CNC phenotype remains unknown.

Since CNC may cause numerous clinical manifestations, including skin, nerve sheath and cardiac tumours (thromboembolic events related to atrial myxoma are a common cause of death), these patients need very careful and frequent monitoring. Given the association with pituitary tumourigenesis, this should include annual pituitary hormone profiling and MRI and very close monitoring of growth curves in children.

PITUITARY ADENOMAS ASSOCIATED WITH PHAEOCHROMOCYTOMAS OR PARAGANGLIOMAS

Over 70 patients have now been described in the published literature who have presented with both a pituitary adenoma and a phaeochromocytoma (phaeo) or paraganglioma (PGL).

Historically, it was assumed that the combination of pituitary adenoma with phaeo/PGL was either an unusual coincidence or a rare manifestation of MEN-1. In fact, of these combination cases thus far described, 30% have had mutations identified in genes already known to predispose to either pituitary tumours or phaeo/PGL [23]. The question remains as to whether the genetic mutations known to predispose to either pituitary adenoma or phaeo/PGL also contribute to the formation of the other.

There is recent evidence to suggest that the classical phaeo/PGL-predisposing genes do indeed have a role in pituitary tumourigenesis, leading to the naming of a new syndrome in 2015 called the 3 PAs [24]. Mutations in any of the four genes encoding the succinate dehydrogenase (SDH) complex subunits A, B, C and D are well described to result in hereditary phaeo/PGL (*SDHx, SDHA, SDHB, SDHC, SDHD*). SDH is part of both the tricarboxylic acid (TCA) cycle and the electron transport chain. Its involvement in the pathogenesis of phaeo/PGL is incompletely understood, but seems to relate to succinate accumulation and mitochondrial abnormalities producing a state of tissue pseudohypoxia. The largest cohort to date of 8 patients with *SDHx* mutations and both phaeo/PGL and pituitary adenomas was published in 2015 [25]. Interestingly, it was shown that the pituitary adenomas in this cohort have a unique and specific histological phenotype characterised by intracytoplasmic vacuoles, the significance of which remains to be elucidated. In the same report, 4 cases of patients with MEN-1 presenting with both phaeo/PGL and pituitary adenomas were also described. Intriguingly, menin staining was absent in the phaeo samples, suggesting a role in the pathogenicity of this rare association.

FAMILIAL ISOLATED PITUITARY ADENOMAS

Familial pituitary tumours that are not associated with MEN 1 or 4 and CNC have been united under the term FIPA [26]. FIPA is a clinical diagnosis essentially characterised by the presence of a pituitary adenoma in more than one family member. It is an autosomal dominant disease with incomplete penetrance. Such families can be divided into two distinct groups according to genetic and phenotypic features. Around 20% of FIPA cases are found to have a mutation in the aryl-hydrocarbon receptor-interacting protein (AIP) gene [27,28]. This group are characterised by young onset, aggressive and treatment-resistant somatotroph or lactotroph macroadenomas [29,30]. The remaining group of FIPA patients, in whom no causative genes have as yet been identified, have a more varied phenotype (although still tend to present with younger onset and larger tumours than sporadic cases).

AIP mutation–positive FIPA

The majority of AIP mutation–positive FIPA patients present in early life, with a mean age of diagnosis around 22 years, ranging from 6 years to 74 years. In fact, 20% of children presenting with a pituitary adenoma are found to harbour this mutation [31]. This falls to 3% of all (apparently sporadic) cases of pituitary adenomas diagnosed in patients under the age of 40 years in a recent prospective study of 127 consecutive patients [32].

Over 65% of AIP mutation–positive pituitary tumours occur in males although there are otherwise no distinguishing clinical features between male and female patients. The mutation is also associated with a greater predilection for somatotroph adenomas (which occur in 40–50% of cases). This, in combination with a tendency for younger onset, explains why pituitary gigantism is well recognised in FIPA kindred [33]. Mixed GH and prolactin or prolactin-secreting macroadenomas are also particularly common in AIP mutation–positive patients, although NFPAs and TSHomas have also all been described [34]. Typically, the somatotroph and lactotroph adenomas that occur in AIP mutation-positive FIPA patients grow aggressively. They tend to belong to the sparsely-granulated subtype and respond poorly to somatostatin analogue or dopamine agonist therapy [35]. For these reasons, such patients require repeated surgery and radiotherapy more often than patients with sporadic pituitary adenomas, and in addition pituitary apoplexy seems to be more common in this cohort.

AIP has been shown to function as a tumour suppressor gene. More than 70 different mutations have been described to date, including a few common (hotspot) mutations (e.g. p.R304X in 35 patients and p.Q14X in 19 patients), most of which lead to a truncated and dysfunctional protein, although one example of an AIP promoter mutation has also been described [18,31]. There have been a number of interesting founder effects described in Finland, Northern Ireland and Italy, some reaching back many centuries [28,36,37]. Families with AIP mutations have a significantly higher number of affected members (3.2 ± 1.8 cases) than AIP mutation-negative FIPA families (2.2 ± 0.4 cases) [26]. However, the level of penetrance of the AIP mutation is quite difficult to establish in the absence of full genetic and clinical data for these families. Furthermore, different mutations may be associated with different levels of penetrance, which ranges across families from 10–80%, probably averaging around 30%. There are also a number of cases of AIP mutations identified in patients without a family history, which could be the result of variations in penetrance or lack of information about the family. To date, a de novo AIP mutation has been described once. All identified mutations have been germline and there is no reported incidence of a somatic AIP mutation in either FIPA or sporadic cases of pituitary adenoma [38]. Furthermore, no genotype–phenotype correlation for age of onset, tumour type or level of penetrance has been established in AIP mutation-positive FIPA.

As with other genetic causes of pituitary tumourigenesis, the function and contribution of the AIP gene product to the molecular mechanism of pituitary adenoma formation remains to be fully elucidated. Novel AIP mouse knockout models have been helpful. Homozygous AIP-/- is embryonically lethal due to multiple structural cardiac deformities [39]. Heterozygous AIP+/– mice are highly prone to pituitary adenomas, with complete penetrance of this effect after 1 year of age. AIP immunohistochemistry of the tumours in these mouse models confirm biallelic inactivation of AIP, which supports its effects as a tumour suppressor gene. Mirroring the human syndrome associated with this mutation, the affected mice develop mainly somatotropinomas (88%), although mixed GH/prolactin, prolactinomas and ACTH-positive adenomas are also detected [40].

AIP is considered to be ubiquitously expressed, albeit to varying degrees among different tissues. In normal pituitary, the AIP protein is expressed in somatotrophs and lactotrophs, where it associates with cytoplasmic secretory vesicles. AIP is expressed in all sporadic pituitary adenomas. In somatotropinomas it specifically colocalises with GH in secretory vesicles, as in normal somatotrophs, whereas in sporadic prolactinomas, corticotropinomas and NFPAs, AIP localises to the cytoplasm [30].

AIP has been shown to interact with multiple cellular proteins and therefore has the potential to interfere with a wide spectrum of cellular and environmental signals [41]. The best-characterised AIP binding partner is the dioxin receptor, also known as AHR [42-44]. AIP is involved in the cytoplasmic retention of AHR and decreases its proteosomal degradation. AHR is a ligand-activated transcription factor which translocates to the nucleus and regulates the transcription of detoxification enzymes that are necessary for the clearance of environmental contaminants such as 2,3,7,8-tetrachlorodibenzo-p-dioxin and polycyclic aromatic hydrocarbons [45]. Interestingly, immunostaining reveals that AHR complexes are significantly reduced in human AIP-associated tumours. Down-regulation of AHR in AIP mutation-positive adenomas may lead to aberrant expression of its target response genes. It has been proposed that the increased prevalence of acromegaly that is observed in highly industrial areas may be related to the effects of pollutants promoting pituitary tumorigenesis [46]. However, in the Seveso population in Italy, after a severe 2,3,7,8-tetrachlorodibenzo-p-dioxin exposure accident in 1976, no statistically significant increase in the prevalence of pituitary tumours was found in a study published 32 years later [47].

Other groups have focussed on trying to understand the basis for the reduced response to somatostatin analogues in acromegalic FIPA patients. Chahal et al. showed that somatostatin receptor expression in FIPA pituitary tumours was not reduced (in fact there was a trend for upregulation of somatostatin 2 and 5 receptor expression). Instead they found that the zinc finger transcription factor *ZAC1* may be involved [48]. *ZAC1* is suggested to be a tumour suppressor gene which induces G1 cell cycle arrest. It is highly expressed in normal pituitary but is down-regulated in pituitary adenomas and it had also been shown that the somatostatin analogue octreotide exerts its antiproliferative action through the up-regulation of *ZAC1* [49,50]. Chahal et al. confirmed that AIP expression is increased in sporadic pituitary tumours from patients previously treated with somatostatin analogues before surgery and that in-vitro AIP knockdown reduced *ZAC1* levels too. Taken together these results suggest that the action of somatostatin analogues on somatotroph tumours is at least partly mediated via AIP effects on *ZAC1*. To date no equivalent studies have been performed on FIPA prolactinomas and dopamine agonists.

In conclusion, the past decade has witnessed great advances in our understanding of the familial pituitary tumour syndrome that occurs in the setting of the AIP mutation. In line with this, the largest research groups involved in clinically phenotyping these kindred are moving towards the establishment of formal guidelines for screening for this mutation. Current suggestions include screening for AIP gene mutations in all patients with FIPA (i.e. patients with a family history of pituitary adenoma), paediatric-onset pituitary adenoma and in patients with acromegaly or a macroprolactinoma before the age of 30 years [31]. This type of screening of AIP mutation positive subjects has been shown to result in early diagnosis and treatment of otherwise possibly devastating, large, and often rapidly growing adenomas. Follow up and monitoring guidance for AIP-mutation carriers without pituitary disease or with small microadenomas is also not yet codified, but should undoubtedly involve a centre with specialist expertise.

AIP mutation–negative cases

A combined analysis of the published results on FIPA cohorts shows that a total of 211 FIPA families have been described in a manner that permits data analysis [26]. Of these, 169 families (80.0%) do not harbour a detectable *AIP* mutation. The total cohort of 211 FIPA families can also be subdivided into homogenous families (that is where the index and related cases have the same pituitary tumour type – 60.2%) and 84 heterogeneous families. There is a higher proportion of *AIP* mutation positivity among homogeneous FIPA families (22.8%) as compared with heterogeneous FIPA kindreds (16.7%).

Indeed, *AIP* mutation–negative FIPA families generally have a more varied clinical phenotype – possibly because they represent a genotypically-mixed group of a number of different, as yet unidentified mutations. Overall, affected patients present at an older age (mean around 40 years, range 12–73 years old) compared with *AIP*-positive patients although they also tend to have more aggressive tumours than sporadic cases, usually presenting with macroadenomas that are either NFPAs, GH-secreting or prolactinomas [26]. Penetrance is probably lower than in *AIP* mutation–positive patients. Interestingly, Cushing's disease (CD) is virtually never found in FIPA. In fact, none of familial pituitary tumour syndromes are particularly associated with ACTH-producing adenoma, pointing towards an acquired rather than a germline genetic basis for CD [51].

Guidelines for how to clinically monitor *AIP*-negative FIPA patients are even more difficult to establish than for other forms of familial pituitary tumour syndromes due to the lack of causative genes that may confer information about natural history. It is generally accepted that their follow-up should be the same as for patients with sporadic tumours. However, a thorough family history is very important to try and identify potentially affected family members as well as gleaning phenotypic information about that particular pedigree. Relatives with clinical symptoms or signs of a pituitary adenoma should be formally tested with imaging and hormone profiles.

CONCLUSION

Familial pituitary tumour syndromes are now a well-recognised clinical entity, recently revitalised with the discovery of the *AIP* gene. Genomic studies of *AIP*-negative FIPA families and the impending widespread clinical application of next-generation sequencing, are likely to discover even more novel loci and causative genes for familial pituitary tumourigenesis. Careful phenotyping in kindred will remain of central importance to contextualise the molecular data generated. Alongside this, there is much work to be done in understanding the role of other endocrine-related neoplasia genes (such as *MEN-1*, *CDKN1b*, *PRKAR1A* and *SDHx*) in pituitary tumourigenesis. A thorough understanding of the molecular mechanisms by which these gene products contribute to normal pituitary function as well as adenoma formation, will have important diagnostic, prognostic and treatment sequelae.

In the meantime, endocrinologists should be aware of the existence and implications of familial pituitary tumour syndromes. Informing family history taking and clinical assessment in this way is necessary to appropriately identify patients with pituitary tumours who should undergo genetic screening and tailored treatment plans.

Key points for clinical practice

- 5% of all pituitary tumours are familial in origin.
- The most common examples are pituitary tumours associated with the MEN-1 syndrome (usually prolactinomas, caused by a mutation in the gene encoding for menin) or FIPA (often aggressive somatotropinomas and associated with a mutation in the AIP gene in 20% of cases).
- Overall, only a minority of causative gene mutations for such tumours have been identified. Widespread use of genetic screening in unselected patients with sporadic pituitary tumours is therefore not indicated.
- A thorough family history is important when assessing any patient with a pituitary tumour. Other markers of a possible germline mutation driving the pituitary tumourigenesis are young patients with aggressive, large or treatment-unresponsive tumours.

REFERENCES

1.   Aflorei ED, Korbonits M. Epidemiology and etiopathogenesis of pituitary adenomas. J Neurooncol 2014; 117:379–394.
2.   Lloyd RV, Kovacs K, Young WF Jr., et al. Pituitary tumours: introduction. In: DeLellis RA, Lloyd RV, Heitz PU and Eng C (Eds). World Hearth Organization Classification of Tumours: Pathology and Genetics of Tumours of Endocrine Organs. Lyon, Paris: IARC Press, 2004.
3.   Thakker RV, Multiple endocrine neoplasia – syndromes of the twentieth century. J Clin Endocrinol Metab 1998; 83:2617–2620.
4.   Thakker RV, Newey PJ, Walls GV, et al. Clinical practice guidelines for multiple endocrine neoplasia type 1 (MEN1). J Clin Endocrinol Metab 2012; 97:2990–3011.
5.   de Laat JM, Dekkers OM, Pieterman CR, et al. Long-Term Natural Course of Pituitary Tumors in Patients With MEN1: Results From the DutchMEN1 Study Group (DMSG). J Clin Endocrinol Metab 2015; 100:3288–3296.
6.   Chandrasekharappa SC, Guru SC, Manickam P, et al. Positional cloning of the gene for multiple endocrine neoplasia-type 1. Science 1997; 276:404–407.
7.   Yang Y, Hua X. In search of tumor suppressing functions of menin. Mol Cell Endocrinol 2007; 265–266:34–41.
8.   Birla SP, P Jyotsna V, Singla R, Tripathi M, Sharma A. Impact of a novel 14 bp MEN1 deletion in a patient with hyperparathyroidism and gastrinoma. Endocrinol Diabetes Metab Case Rep 2015; 2015:150011.
9.   Fujiya A, Kato M, Shibata T, Sobajima H. VIPoma with multiple endocrine neoplasia type 1 identified as an atypical gene mutation. BMJ Case Rep 2015.
10. Jyotsna VP, Malik E, Birla S, Sharma A. Novel MEN 1 gene findings in rare sporadic insulinoma – a case control study. BMC Endocr Disord 2015; 15:44.
11. Ning Z, Wang O, Meng X, et al. MEN1 c.8251G> A mutation in a family with multiple endocrine neoplasia type 1: A case report. Mol Med Rep 2015; 12:6152–6156.
12. Remde H, Kaminsky E, Werner M, Quinkler M. A patient with novel mutations causing MEN1 and hereditary multiple osteochondroma. Endocrinol Diabetes Metab Case Rep, 2015. Published online doi: 10.1530/EDM-14-0120.
13. Lemos MC, Thakker RV. Multiple endocrine neoplasia type 1 (MEN1): analysis of 1336 mutations reported in the first decade following identification of the gene. Hum Mutat 2008; 29:22–32.
14. Thevenon J, Bourredjem A, Faivre L, et al. Unraveling the intrafamilial correlations and heritability of tumor types in MEN1: a Groupe d'etude des Tumeurs Endocrines study. Eur J Endocrinol 2015; 173:819–826.
15. Pellegata NS, Quintanilla-Martinez L, Siggelkow H, et al. Germ-line mutations in p27Kip1 cause a multiple endocrine neoplasia syndrome in rats and humans. Proc Natl Acad Sci USA 2006; 103:15558–15563.
16. Georgitsi M, Raitila A, Karhu A, et al. Germline CDKN1B/p27Kip1 mutation in multiple endocrine neoplasia. J Clin Endocrinol Metab 2007; 92:3321–3325.
17. Tichomirowa MA, Lee M, Barlier A, et al. Cyclin-dependent kinase inhibitor 1B (CDKN1B) gene variants in AIP mutation-negative familial isolated pituitary adenoma kindreds. Endocr Relat Cancer 2012; 19:233–241.
18. Igreja S, Chahal HS, Akker SA, et al. Assessment of p27 (cyclin-dependent kinase inhibitor 1B) and aryl hydrocarbon receptor-interacting protein (AIP) genes in multiple endocrine neoplasia (MEN1) syndrome patients without any detectable MEN1 gene mutations. Clin Endocrinol (Oxf) 2009; 70:259–264.
19. Correa RP. Salpea, Stratakis CA. Carney complex: an update. Eur J Endocrinol 2015; 173:M85–97.
20. Bertherat J, Horvath A, Groussin L, et al. Mutations in regulatory subunit type 1A of cyclic adenosine 5'-monophosphate-dependent protein kinase (PRKAR1A): phenotype analysis in 353 patients and 80 different genotypes. J Clin Endocrinol Metab 2009; 94:2085–2091.
21. Horvath A, Bertherat J, Groussin L, et al. Mutations and polymorphisms in the gene encoding regulatory subunit type 1-alpha of protein kinase A (PRKAR1A): an update. Hum Mutat 2010; 31:369–379.
22. Stratakis CA, Carney JA, Lin JP, et al. Carney complex, a familial multiple neoplasia and lentiginosis syndrome. Analysis of 11 kindreds and linkage to the short arm of chromosome 2. J Clin Invest 1996; 97:699–705.
23. O'Toole SM, Dénes J, Robledo M, Stratakis CA, Korbonits M. 15 YEARS OF PARAGANGLIOMA: The association of pituitary adenomas and phaeochromocytomas or paragangliomas. Endocr Relat Cancer 2015; 22:T105–122.
24. Xekouki P, Szarek E, Bullova P, et al. Pituitary adenoma with paraganglioma/pheochromocytoma (3PAs) and succinate dehydrogenase defects in humans and mice. J Clin Endocrinol Metab 2015; 100:E710–719.

25. Denes J, Swords F, Rattenberry E, et al. Heterogeneous genetic background of the association of pheochromocytoma/paraganglioma and pituitary adenoma: results from a large patient cohort. J Clin Endocrinol Metab 2015; 100:E531–541.

26. Beckers A, Aaltonen LA, Daly AF, Karhu A. Familial isolated pituitary adenomas (FIPA) and the pituitary adenoma predisposition due to mutations in the aryl hydrocarbon receptor interacting protein (AIP) gene. Endocr Rev 2013; 34:239–277.

27. Daly AF, Vanbellinghen JF, Khoo SK, et al. Aryl hydrocarbon receptor-interacting protein gene mutations in familial isolated pituitary adenomas: analysis in 73 families. J Clin Endocrinol Metab 2007; 92:1891–1896.

28. Vierimaa O, Georgitsi M, Lehtonen R, et al. Pituitary adenoma predisposition caused by germline mutations in the AIP gene. Science 2006; 312:1228–1230.

29. Williams F, Hunter S, Bradley L, et al. Clinical experience in the screening and management of a large kindred with familial isolated pituitary adenoma due to an aryl hydrocarbon receptor interacting protein (AIP) mutation. J Clin Endocrinol Metab 2014; 99:1122–1131.

30. Leontiou CA, Gueorguiev M, van der Spuy J, et al. The role of the aryl hydrocarbon receptor-interacting protein gene in familial and sporadic pituitary adenomas. J Clin Endocrinol Metab 2008; 93:2390–2401.

31. Korbonits M, Storr H, Kumar AV. Familial pituitary adenomas – who should be tested for AIP mutations? Clin Endocrinol (Oxf) 2012; 77:351–356.

32. Preda V, Korbonits M, Cudlip S, Karavitaki N, Grossman AB. Low rate of germline AIP mutations in patients with apparently sporadic pituitary adenomas before the age of 40: a single-centre adult cohort. Eur J Endocrinol 2014; 171:659–666.

33. Rostomyan L, Daly AF, Petrossians P, et al. Clinical and genetic characterization of pituitary gigantism: an international collaborative study in 208 patients. Endocr Relat Cancer 2015; 22:745–757.

34. Chahal HS, Chapple JP, Frohman LA, Grossman AB, Korbonits M. Clinical, genetic and molecular characterization of patients with familial isolated pituitary adenomas (FIPA). Trends Endocrinol Metab 2010; 21:419–427.

35. Daly AF, Tichomirowa MA, Petrossians P, et al. Clinical characteristics and therapeutic responses in patients with germ-line AIP mutations and pituitary adenomas: an international collaborative study. J Clin Endocrinol Metab 2010; 95:E373–383.

36. Chahal HS, Stals K, Unterländer M, et al. AIP mutation in pituitary adenomas in the 18th century and today. N Engl J Med 2011; 364:43–50.

37. Occhi G, Jaffrain-Rea ML, Trivellin G, et al. The R304X mutation of the aryl hydrocarbon receptor interacting protein gene in familial isolated pituitary adenomas: Mutational hot-spot or founder effect? J Endocrinol Invest 2010; 33:800–805.

38. Stratakis CA, Tichomirowa MA, Boikos S, et al. The role of germline AIP, MEN1, PRKAR1A, CDKN1B and CDKN2C mutations in causing pituitary adenomas in a large cohort of children, adolescents, and patients with genetic syndromes. Clin Genet 2010; 78:457–463.

39. Lin BC, Sullivan R, Lee Y, et al. Deletion of the aryl hydrocarbon receptor-associated protein 9 leads to cardiac malformation and embryonic lethality. J Biol Chem 2007; 282:35924–35932.

40. Raitila A, Lehtonen HJ, Arola J, et al. Mice with inactivation of aryl hydrocarbon receptor-interacting protein (AIP) display complete penetrance of pituitary adenomas with aberrant ARNT expression. Am J Pathol 2010; 177:1969–1976.

41. Trivellin G, Butz H, Delhove J, et al. MicroRNA miR-107 is overexpressed in pituitary adenomas and inhibits the expression of aryl hydrocarbon receptor-interacting protein in vitro. Am J Physiol Endocrinol Metab 2012; 303:E708–719.

42. Petrulis JR, Perdew GH. The role of chaperone proteins in the aryl hydrocarbon receptor core complex. Chem Biol Interact 2002; 141:25–40.

43. Pollenz RS, Dougherty EJ. Redefining the role of the endogenous XAP2 and C-terminal hsp70-interacting protein on the endogenous Ah receptors expressed in mouse and rat cell lines. J Biol Chem 2005; 280:33346–33356.

44. Heliovaara E, Raitila A, Launonen V, et al. The expression of AIP-related molecules in elucidation of cellular pathways in pituitary adenomas. Am J Pathol 2009; 175:2501–2507.

45. Ramadoss P, Perdew GH. The transactivation domain of the Ah receptor is a key determinant of cellular localization and ligand-independent nucleocytoplasmic shuttling properties. Biochemistry 2005; 44:11148–11159.

46. Cannavo S, Ferraù F, Ragonese M, et al. Increased prevalence of acromegaly in a highly polluted area. Eur J Endocrinol 2010; 163:509–513.

47. Pesatori AC, Baccarelli A, Consonni D, et al. Aryl hydrocarbon receptor-interacting protein and pituitary adenomas: a population-based study on subjects exposed to dioxin after the Seveso, Italy, accident. Eur J Endocrinol 2008; 159:699–703.

48. Chahal HS, Trivellin G, Leontiou CA, et al. Somatostatin analogs modulate AIP in somatotroph adenomas: the role of the ZAC1 pathway. J Clin Endocrinol Metab 2012; 97:E1411–420.

49. Theodoropoulou M, Zhang J, Laupheimer S, et al. Octreotide, a somatostatin analogue, mediates its antiproliferative action in pituitary tumor cells by altering phosphatidylinositol 3-kinase signaling and inducing ZAC1 expression. Cancer Res 2006; 66:1576–1582.

50. Theodoropoulou M, Tichomirowa MA, Sievers C, et al. Tumor ZAC1 expression is associated with the response to somatostatin analog therapy in patients with acromegaly. Int J Cancer 2009; 125:2122–1226.

51. Theodoropoulou M, Reincke M, Fassnacht M, Komada M. Decoding the genetic basis of Cushing's disease: USP8 in the spotlight. Eur J Endocrinol 2015; 173:M73–83.

Chapter 2

Treatments for acromegaly

Saira Hameed, Niamh Martin

INTRODUCTION

Acromegaly, the clinical manifestation of pathological growth hormone (GH) and insulin-like growth factor-1 (IGF-1) excess, is a rare but important endocrinopathy. The incidence of acromegaly is 2.9 cases per million with a prevalence of 56.5 cases per million. Acromegaly is more commonly diagnosed in women (70% of cases), with a mean age at diagnosis of 46 years. Acromegaly is almost invariably caused by a pituitary adenoma, although rare cases can arise from a pituitary adenocarcinoma or from ectopic secretion of growth hormone releasing hormone (GHRH) or rarely GH itself. Treatment of acromegaly aims to normalise GH and IGF-1 levels, reduce the mass effect of the tumour, manage the complications and achieve optimal health related quality of life.

Within a generation, medical treatment options have come to the fore in the treatment of acromegaly and now sit alongside surgery and radiotherapy in terms of efficacy and long term outcomes. There are three classes of drug that are widely used in clinical practice, somatostatin analogues (SSAs), dopamine receptor agonists and the GH receptor antagonist pegvisomant. In addition, traditional chemotherapy agents such as temozolamide are emerging as treatment for selected highly aggressive tumours and next generation agents such as oral SSAs are also under development. Lastly, the use of molecular biology and histopathology to characterise the phenotype of the tumour has the potential to guide medical treatment decisions in the future.

SOMATOSTATIN ANALOGUES

Somatotroph adenomas express somatostatin receptors (SSTR) which exist as 5 subtypes named SSTR1 to SSTR5. Somatostatin is a hypothalamic peptide that acts on somatotrophs to inhibit GH secretion. The endogenous effect of somatostatin is mimicked by the SSAs octreotide and lanreotide which are both also available as long acting formulations. SSAs can be used as a first line treatment for acromegaly resulting in normalisation of circulating GH and IGF-1 in about a third of patients [1,2] and tumour shrinkage in up to 50% of patients, normally within months [3,4] although a recent meta-analysis failed to find a benefit from SSA pre-treatment prior to surgery [5].

Niamh Martin MBChB PhD FRCP, Imperial Centre for Endocrinology, Charing Cross Hospital, London, UK. Email: n.martin@imperial.ac.uk (for correspondence).

Saira Hameed MA (Oxon) MRCP PhD, Imperial Centre for Endocrinology, Charing Cross Hospital, London, UK.

In clinical practice, the most commonly used SSAs are long-acting octreotide and lanreotide which appear to have similar outcomes in terms of symptom control [6]. These long-acting preparations act predominantly at SSTR2, which is important because tumours differ in their expression profile of SSTRs with 52% of somatotroph adenomas being SSTR5 dominant and 39% SSTR2 dominant [7]. In clinical studies there is a positive correlation between SSTR2 expression and percentage decrease in GH and IGF-1 after starting treatment with octreotide long-acting repeatable (LAR) [7]. This opens up the possibility that classification of tumours by SSTR expression could hold a predictive value for response to medical therapy. In addition, newer SSAs are emerging which show selectivity at additional SSTRs, for example somatoprim which has a high affinity for SSTR3, in addition to SSTR2 and SSTR5. In pre-clinical work, when applied to cultures of somatotroph adenoma cells, all of which were found to express SSTR3, somatoprim produced greater suppression of GH secretion than octreotide [8]. It is noteworthy that in addition to differing patterns of SSTR subtype expression, SSTR mutations have been identified in some tumours, for example mutation of the SSTR5 receptor, which could explain SSA treatment resistance in some patients [9].

The histological appearance of the tumour is also a useful marker for predicting response to medical therapy. On electron microscopy, somatotroph adenomas appear to be either densely or sparsely granulated, with densely-granulated expressing SSTR2 more highly than sparsely-granulated adenomas [10]. Consistent with this, it has been reported that patients with densely-granulated adenomas are more likely to achieve a normalisation of GH and IGF-1 when treated with SSAs [11].

Pasireotide is a high-affinity SSA that targets multiple SSTRs [12] with an increased affinity for the SSTR5 compared to octreotide and lanreotide. In comparison to octreotide LAR, pasireotide LAR has been shown to achieve superior biochemical control in both treatment-naïve and post-operative acromegaly patients over 12 months of treatment [13], although concerns have been raised about the dose of octreotide LAR used. A significant drawback to the use of pasireotide is the high incidence of new cases of hyperglycaemia or deterioration of pre-existing cases, with patients frequently requiring initiation of or intensification of glucose-lowering medication [13].

A drawback of the currently available SSAs is that they must be injected which is an issue for some patients. Recently, an oral octreotide preparation has been developed. The route of delivery has proved possible because the carrier capsule has properties, known as transient permeability enhancer technology, which induces transient opening of tight junctions of the intestinal epithelium, allowing the passage of the drug from the gut into the systemic circulation [14]. In preliminary studies, oral octreotide achieved biochemical control of acromegaly in 65% of subjects and this was maintained for up to 13 months [15]. Adverse effects were similar to those reported for injectable SSAs. Approval for use from regulatory authorities both in Europe and the US is awaited.

DOPAMINE AGONISTS

The neuropeptide dopamine inhibits GH release through its interaction with dopamine (D2) receptors which are expressed on somatotrophs. Somatotroph adenomas also express dopamine receptors and dopamine agonists are therefore used to reduce the GH burden either alone or in combination with another drug, usually an SSA. In practice, the most commonly used dopamine agonist is the ergot derivative cabergoline. When used alone, cabergoline normalises IGF-1 in 34% of patients either as first line treatment or following surgery and/or radiotherapy, a figure which rises to 50% with the addition of an SSA [16]. Analysis of responders shows that those with milder disease (IGF-1 less than twice upper limit of normal) are more likely to benefit from cabergoline than those with a heavier disease burden.

Reports of cardiac valve regurgitation in patients with Parkinson's disease treated with dopamine agonists [17] created alarm in the endocrine community because of the widespread use of dopamine agonists in the treatment of both acromegaly and hyperprolactinaemia. Subsequent studies have concluded that dopamine agonists can be safely used to treat both acromegaly and hyperprolactinaemia, without causing cardiac valvular dysfunction [18,19]. It was determined that the difference between endocrine and neurology outcomes was likely to be explained by the administered dose, typically many orders of magnitude higher when used to treat Parkinson's disease. On the whole cabergoline is well tolerated although some patients experience nausea and postural dizziness which can be ameliorated by slow dose up-titration. Dopamine agonists can also negatively affect mood and care should be exercised in prescribing these drugs to patients currently or previously known to have a mood disorder, e.g. depression.

GROWTH HORMONE RECEPTOR ANTAGONISTS – PEGVISOMANT

Pegvisomant, an injected GH receptor antagonist, has now been in clinical use for over a decade. Its use is usually restricted to patients who have failed to achieve disease control with SSAs and/or dopamine agonists or following surgery. Because pegvisomant acts at the level of the GH receptor, GH levels cannot be used clinically to measure disease activity and treatment response is therefore guided by symptomatology and by circulating IGF-1. The ACROSTUDY was established in 2004 as an international surveillance trial examining post-marketing safety. A report on almost a decade of experience with pegvisomant [20] showed that although two thirds of patients had normal IGF-1 levels after 5 years of treatment, in three quarters of patients there was no change in tumour size on serial MRI. Previously reported concerns relating to abnormalities in liver function tests were not corroborated by the ACROSTUDY. In clinical practice, the key issue relating to pegvisomant use is cost.

TEMOZOLOMIDE

There is a growing interest in the use of the chemotherapy agent temozolamide for the treatment of aggressive pituitary tumours. Temozolamide is an oral alkylating agent which has been found to have variable success in the treatment of pituitary carcinomas and some aggressive adenomas. Temozolamide has been widely used in the treatment of glioblastoma and studies on cell lines from these tumours suggest that the efficacy of this agent may in part be due to the patient's O^6-methylguanine-DNA methyltransferase (MGMT; a DNA repair protein) status [21,22]. Studies have consistently reported that tumours with a high level of MGMT expression on immunohistochemistry respond poorly in comparison to those with low MGMT, a finding which has the potential to inform clinical decision making. To date, experience of temozolamide for the treatment of aggressive GH adenomas or carcinomas is limited to three reported case series comprising a total of 21 patients in whom tumour control was achieved in 50% [22].

CONCLUSION

Over a hundred years since the term 'acromegaly' was first coined, the management of this condition remains complex and challenging. Most clinicians with experience of the disease will agree that no two patients with acromegaly are quite the same. Therefore, where published results are quoted above, it is important to note that these are based on a cohort rather than on any individual patient and that in practice, a myriad of patient and tumour factors determine symptomatology and response to treatment. It is therefore essential that patients with suspected or confirmed acromegaly are managed within a multi-disciplinary team in a dedicated pituitary centre. In addition, it is noteworthy that a major cause of morbidity in acromegaly is the associated cardiovascular disease burden and therefore optimisation of cardiovascular risk factors, for example blood pressure and glycaemic control plays a synchronous role with the control of GH burden. The art of using medical therapies for the management of acromegaly continues to evolve and new agents will add to the currently available armoury. In addition, phenotyping of tumours by their receptor expression, mutation patterns, histological appearance or intracellular machinery is likely to emerge as a valuable tool to guide the choice of treatment and to predict treatment response in the future.

Key points for clinical practice

- Acromegaly is a rare and clinically challenging endocrinopathy which should be managed in a specialist multi-disciplinary pituitary centre.

- Three main classes of drug are used to manage acromegaly. Two exploit somatotroph adenoma receptor expression. Both somatostatin and dopamine inhibit GH secretion acting through somatostatin and dopamine receptors respectively, and somatostain analogues and dopamine agonists are therefore used to control GH burden. A third class of drug, the GH receptor antagonist pegvisomant, achieves biochemical control of the disease, but its clinical use is limited by its high cost.

- Patients show a heterogeneous response to medical treatments for acromegaly. In the future tumour molecular and histopathological sub-typing may allow for efficacious individualised treatment regimens.

REFERENCES

1. Giustina A, Chanson P, Bronstein MD. A consensus on criteria for cure of acromegaly. J Clin Endocrinol Metab 2010; 95:3141–3148.
2. Ben-Shlomo A, Melmed S. Somatostatin agonists for treatment of acromegaly. Mol Cell Endocrinol 2008; 286:192–198.
3. Giustina A, Mazziotti G, Torri V, et al. Meta-analysis on the effects of octreotide on tumor mass in acromegaly. PLoS One 2012; 7:e36411.
4. Lamberts SW, Krenning EP, Reubi JC. The role of somatostatin and its analogs in the diagnosis and treatment of tumors. Endocr Rev 1991; 12:450–482.
5. Fougner SL, Bollerslev J, Svartberg J, et al. Preoperative octreotide treatment of acromegaly: long-term results of a randomised controlled trial. Eur J Endocrinol 2014; 171:229–235.
6. Murray RD, Melmed S. A critical analysis of clinically available somatostatin analog formulations for therapy of acromegaly. J Clin Endocrinol Metab 2008; 93:2957–2968.

7. Taboada GF, Luque RM, Bastos W, et al. Quantitative analysis of somatostatin receptor subtype (SSTR1-5) gene expression levels in somatotropinomas and non-functioning pituitary adenomas. Eur J Endocrinol 2007; 156:65–74.

8. Plockinger U, Hoffmann U, Geese M, et al. DG3173 (somatoprim), a unique somatostatin receptor subtypes 2-, 4- and 5-selective analogue, effectively reduces GH secretion in human GH-secreting pituitary adenomas even in Octreotide non-responsive tumours. Eur J Endocrinol 2012; 166:223–234.

9. Ballare E, Persani L, Lania AG, et al. Mutation of somatostatin receptor type 5 in an acromegalic patient resistant to somatostatin analog treatment. J Clin Endocrinol Metab 2001; 86:3809–3814.

10. Kato M, Inoshita N, Sugiyama T, et al. Differential expression of genes related to drug responsiveness between sparsely and densely granulated somatotroph adenomas. Endocr J 2012; 59:221–228.

11. Bhayana S, Booth GL, Asa SL, Kovacs K, Ezzat S. The implication of somatotroph adenoma phenotype to somatostatin analog responsiveness in acromegaly. J Clin Endocrinol Metab 2005; 90:6290–6295.

12. Bruns C, Lewis I, Briner U, Meno-Tetang G, Weckbecker G. SOM230: a novel somatostatin peptidomimetic with broad somatotropin release inhibiting factor (SRIF) receptor binding and a unique antisecretory profile. Eur J Endocrinol 2002; 146:707–716.

13. Colao A, Bronstein MD, Freda P, et al. Pasireotide versus octreotide in acromegaly: a head-to-head superiority study. J Clin Endocrinol Metab 2014; 99:791–799.

14. Tuvia S, Pelled D, Marom K, et al. A novel suspension formulation enhances intestinal absorption of macromolecules via transient and reversible transport mechanisms. Pharm Res 2014; 31:2010–2021.

15. Melmed S, Popovic V, Bidlingmaier M, et al. Safety and efficacy of oral octreotide in acromegaly: results of a multicenter phase III trial. J Clin Endocrinol Metab 2015; 100:1699–1708.

16. Sandret L, Maison P, Chanson P. Place of cabergoline in acromegaly: a meta-analysis. J Clin Endocrinol Metab 2011; 96:1327–1335.

17. Schade R, Andersohn F, Suissa S, Haverkamp W, Garbe E. Dopamine agonists and the risk of cardiac-valve regurgitation. N Engl J Med 2007; 356:29–38.

18. Tan T, Cabrita IZ, Hensman D, et al. Assessment of cardiac valve dysfunction in patients receiving cabergoline treatment for hyperprolactinaemia. Clin Endocrinol (Oxf) 2010; 73:369–374.

19. Maione L, Garcia C, Bouchachi A, et al. No evidence of a detrimental effect of cabergoline therapy on cardiac valves in patients with acromegaly. J Clin Endocrinol Metab 2012; 97:E1714–1719.

20. van der Lely AJ, Biller BM, Brue T, et al. Long-term safety of pegvisomant in patients with acromegaly: comprehensive review of 1288 subjects in ACROSTUDY. J Clin Endocrinol Metab 2012; 97:1589–1597.

21. Cao VT, Jung TY, Jung S, et al. The correlation and prognostic significance of MGMT promoter methylation and MGMT protein in glioblastomas. Neurosurgery 2009; 65:866–875.

22. Raverot G, Castinetti F, Jouanneau E, et al. Pituitary carcinomas and aggressive pituitary tumours: merits and pitfalls of temozolomide treatment. Clin Endocrinol (Oxf) 2012; 76:769–775.

Chapter 3

Update on the diagnosis and management of Cushing's syndrome

Karim Meeran, Monika Reddy

INTRODUCTION

Cushing's syndrome is the conglomeration of signs and symptoms caused by excessive circulating cortisol and is associated with poor quality of life [1,2], morbidity, and increased mortality [3,4,5]. The hypothalamic-pituitary axis (HPA) consists of hypothalamic release of corticotrophin-releasing hormone (CRH) which stimulates the synthesis and secretion of adrenocorticotropic hormone (ACTH) from corticotrophs of the anterior pituitary. ACTH stimulates the production and secretion of cortisol from the adrenal cortex (**Figure 3.1**).

In endogenous Cushing's syndrome (the focus of this chapter) high cortisol levels result from either autonomous over-production of cortisol from the adrenal cortex or stimulation by excess ACTH from a pituitary or ectopic tumour. Only rarely does it arise from excess CRH release. The best treatment option is tumour-directed surgical excision, but unsuccessful surgery or contraindications to surgery require initiation of drugs to treat the clinical symptoms associated with hypercortisolaemia. This chapter aims to give an

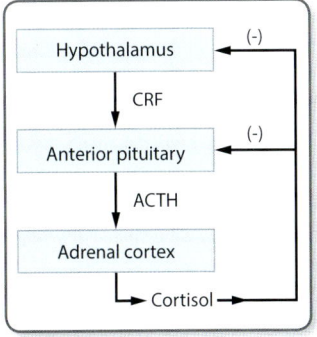

Figure 3.1 Normal hypothalamic-pituitary axis with negative feedback. Cortisol produced in the adrenal cortex will negatively feedback on the hypothalamus and the pituitary and in turn reduce secretion of CRH and ACTH respectively.

Karim Meeran BSc MBBS MD FRCP FRCPath, Department of Diabetes, Endocrinology and Metabolism, Imperial College Healthcare NHS Trust and Imperial College London, UK. Email: k.meeran@imperial.ac.uk (for correspondence).

Monika Reddy MBChB SCE MRCP (Endocrinology & Diabetes) PhD, Department of Diabetes, Endocrinology and Metabolism, Imperial College Healthcare NHS Trust and Imperial College London, UK.

overview of the diagnosis and management of endogenous Cushing's syndrome with some common pitfalls highlighted.

EPIDEMIOLOGY

The prevalence of Cushing's syndrome ranges from 39–79/million. The estimated incidence is 0.2–5.0/million/year [3,6-8]. There is a female-to-male ratio of 3:1 and the median age at diagnosis is 41 years. Approximately 80% of endogenous Cushing's is ACTH-dependent (pituitary or ectopic) and 20% ACTH-independent (primary adrenal) [9].

CLASSIFICATION AND PATHOPHYSIOLOGY OF ENDOGENOUS CUSHING'S SYNDROME

Adrenocorticotrophic hormone dependent (80% of endogenous Cushing's syndrome)

Cushing's disease (60–70%)

Nearly all cases of Cushing's disease are caused by a unilateral pituitary corticotroph adenoma that tends to present in the 3rd-4th decade. Approximately 40% of corticotroph adenomas are not visible on a pituitary magnetic resonance imaging (MRI). Corticotroph hyperplasia rather than adenoma can also cause Cushing's disease, but is very rare. Germline mutations are rare in Cushing's disease but include multiple endocrine neoplasia 1 (MEN-1), aryl-hydrocarbon receptor-interacting protein (AIP) and *CDKN1B* (also known as *p27Kip1*) genes and other cyclin-dependent kinase inhibitor (CDK1) [10]. Somatic mutations in the USP8 deubiquitinase gene in corticotroph adenomas have been shown to cause Cushing's disease via activation of endothelial growth factor receptor signaling [11].

Ectopic adrenocorticotrophic hormone (5–10% of endogenous Cushing's syndrome)

Extrapituitary (ectopic) tumours that secrete ACTH are much less common than Cushing's disease and include benign, occult and malignant neuroendocrine tumours.

Ectopic corticotrophin-releasing hormone

Corticotrophin-releasing hormone tumours leading to excess secretion of ACTH from the pituitary gland are very rare, but include neuroendocrine tumours, phaeochromocytoma and medullary thyroid carcinoma, leading to excess pituitary ACTH secretion.

Pituitary adrenocorticotrophic hormone independent (20–30% of endogenous Cushing's syndrome)

Unilateral adrenal adenomas

These constitute 10–12% of all cases of endogenous Cushing's syndrome and present in the 4th-5th decade. A smaller proportion of unilateral adrenal lesions are malignant and either present in childhood or in the 5th-6th decade and tend to produce a combination of cortisol and androgens.

Bilateral adrenal

Bilateral adrenal lesions are rare and consist of a collection of pathologies including bilateral macronodular and micronodular adrenal hyperplasia, bilateral adenomas and carcinoma.

Primary bilateral nodular adrenal hyperplasia represents less than 2% of all cases of Cushing's syndrome. Excess cortisol secretion from bilateral macronodular adrenal hyperplasia, despite suppressed ACTH levels, was thought to be an autonomous process, but it has been shown that these hyperplastic adrenal glands display abnormal expression of various hormone receptors that are involved in the control of cortisol production [12]. Interestingly, it has also been shown that corticotrophin can be produced within the adrenocortical tissue and act as a local amplifier of the action of these receptors [13].

A host of germline mutations have been associated with unilateral and bilateral nodular hyperplasia [14,15], but the details are beyond the scope of this chapter.

MORBIDITY AND MORTALITY

Hypercortisolaemia is associated with other medical comorbidities including obesity, diabetes, hypertension, cardiovascular disease, cerebrovascular disease and osteoporosis [16-18]. The immunosuppressive effect of hypercortisolaemia also predisposes to opportunistic infections and impairs natural healing processes [16]. Cushing's syndrome also increases the risk of developing thromboembolic disease such as pulmonary embolism and deep vein thrombosis due to the associated hypercoagulable state [19]. Excess and prolonged cortisol exposure on the brain can lead to psychiatric manifestations such as depression and psychosis and to cognitive dysfunction such as impaired memory [20,21].

Screening for Cushing's syndrome as a secondary cause for some of the aforementioned conditions should be considered, particularly when unexplained, i.e. osteoporosis in a young person with no other risk factors.

Successful treatment of Cushing's syndrome and thereby reversing hypercortisolaemia will improve features of certain conditions, such as bone mineral density and cognitive impairment, but may not achieve remission of these co-morbidities [22,23]. The psychological and physical effects of Cushing's syndrome have a negative effect on overall quality of life in people with the condition [16].

The mortality in Cushing's syndrome is increased compared to the general population with most deaths being secondary to cardiovascular disease. The standard mortality ratio (SMR) in Cushing's syndrome has been calculated to be approximately 2.0–4.0 and although the SMR improves after long-term remission it may not return to a normal SMR [3,8,24-26].

CLINICAL SIGNS AND SYMPTOMS

The clinical presentation of Cushing's syndrome is variable as there is a magnitude of associated signs and symptoms (see **Table 3.1**) that are present in normal people and, therefore getting the diagnosis correct can be very challenging. The most discriminatory features include proximal muscle weakness, pigmented-purple striae, plethora and easy bruising [27]. Weight gain is now as prevalent in the normal population as in Cushing's syndrome and is no longer a useful discriminant. As mentioned, prolonged exposure to hypercortisolaemia can lead to co-morbidities such as osteoporosis, cardiovascular

Table 3.1 Clinical features of Cushing's syndrome	
Presenting symptoms	
• Lethargy	• Headache
• Change in mood and cognition	• Generalised swelling
• Abdominal pain	• Recurrent infections
	• Change in menstrual cycle
Signs on clinical examination	
• Purple striae*	• Round face ('moon face')
• Bruising*	• Dorsal fat pad
• Proximal muscle weakness*	• Hirsuitism
• Plethora*	• Hypertension
• Wasting of the extremities	• Thin skin
*Discriminatory features	

disease, thromboembolism, diabetes, psychiatric illness and recurrent illness due to immunosuppression. Individuals with suspected hypercortisolaemia may therefore present to a variety of specialists (e.g orthopaedics, cardiology, gynaecology and neurology) prior to Cushing's syndrome being evaluated as an underlying condition.

INVESTIGATIONS

Initial biochemical screening tests for diagnosis of Cushing's syndrome

Before conducting any biochemical screening exogenous administration of glucocorticoids should be excluded where possible. The endocrine society's clinical practice guideline recommends using two of three screening tests to establish the diagnosis: the 1-mg overnight dexamethasone suppression test, longer-dose dexamethasone suppression test (2 mg/day for 48 h), urinary-free cortisol (UFC) or late night salivary cortisol [28].

Prior to making a decision to perform any biochemical test for establishing the diagnosis it is important to remember that a number of conditions are associated with raised physiological levels of cortisol in the absence of Cushing's syndrome and may therefore result in false positive test results (**Table 3.2**). Pseudo Cushing's refers to physiological over-activity of the HPA axis associated with physical or psychological stress [29]. Pseudo Cushing's syndrome may be seen in patients with anorexia nervosa, depression, alcoholism, obesity and diabetes. If the diagnosis cannot be excluded on clinical grounds then the biochemical screening test should ideally be done once circumstances are optimised, i.e. after treatment of the underlying condition and avoid testing after strenuous exercise or during hospital admission.

The European Endocrine Society highlights the importance of careful clinical evaluation before investigating for Cushing's syndrome and only recommends investigation in the following groups:
1. Those with unusual features for age (e.g. diabetes, hypertension, and osteoporosis)
2. Those with multiple and progressive features, particularly those which are more predictive of Cushing's syndrome
3. Children with decreasing height percentile and increasing weight

Table 3.2 Causes of physiological hypercortisolaemia with or without clinical features	
• Pregnancy • Obesity • Diabetes mellitus • Psychiatric conditions, e.g. depression • Alcohol dependence • Glucocorticoid resistance	• Intense exercise • Malnutrition • Anorexia nervosa • Hypothalamic amenorrhoea • Physical stress, e.g. pain, trauma, surgery • Cortisol-binding globulin excess, e.g. oral contraceptive, PCOS

Table 3.3 Medication that interfere with dexamethasone	
Drugs that impair dexamethasone metabolism by inhibition of CYP 3A4 causing false positive results	
Itraconazole	Fluoxetine
Ritonavir	Diltiazem
Aprepitant/fosaprepitant	Cimetedine
Drugs that accelerate dexamethasone metabolism by induction of CYP3A4 causing false negative/normal results	
Phenobarbitol	Rifampacin
Phenytoin	Rifapentine
Carbamazepine	Ethosuximide
Primidone	Pioglitazone

4. Those with adrenal incidentaloma compatible with adenoma, although this is controversial

Overnight dexamethasone suppression test

This test can be done as an outpatient and involves the patient taking 1 mg of dexamethasone by mouth, between 23:00 h and midnight. The patient then attends for a blood test between 08:00 h and 09:00 h the following morning for measurement of serum cortisol. The overnight dexamethasone suppression test assesses whether glucocorticoid negative feedback is normal. The results are normal if the cortisol is less than 50 nmol/L.

False positives or negative results

False positive results can occur if there is an increase in cortisol-binding globulin (CBG) which increases the total serum cortisol, e.g. in a woman on the oral contraceptive pill or hormone-replacement therapy [30]. Dexamethasone is metabolised by the hepatic *CYP3A4* enzyme complex, which is inhibited or stimulated by many commonly used drugs which may result in false positive results or false negative results respectively (**Table 3.3**).

48-hour low-dose dexamethasone suppression test

This test can be done as outpatient with clear written instructions given to the patient. Patients are informed to take 0.5 mg of dexamethasone at 09:00 h on day 1, then at 6 hourly intervals, i.e. at 09:00 h, 15:00 h, 21:00 h and 03:00 h. The patient then attends for a blood test at 09:00 h on day 2 to measure serum cortisol. The test is negative (i.e. excludes Cushing's syndrome) if the day 2 (48 h) cortisol is less than 50 nmol/L.

The same precautions for avoiding false positives and false negatives should be taken as for the 1-mg overnight dexamethasone suppression test. False positives result in harm to patients who undergo inappropriate surgery.

Urinary-free cortisol

The test involves the patient collecting their urine in a container over 24 hours. The inconvenience associated with this sometimes leads to incomplete collections and it is therefore useful to measure urinary creatinine and the volume of urine. UFC reflects the integrated tissue exposure to free cortisol over 24 hours and so provides a useful perspective on glucocorticoid physiology that gives different information to the overnight and low-dose dexamethasone suppression tests (LDDSTs). This test needs to be repeated at least twice.

False positive and negative results

In those individuals where there is a suspicion of pseudo Cushing's, the overnight and LDDSTs are a better option to avoid false positive results associated with UFC. UFC can give a false negative result when the glomerular filtration rate is low [31] and false positive result if the urine volume is too low [32]. At least two UFC measurement are needed in cases of cyclical Cushing's (intermittent hypercortisolaemia) to avoid false negatives.

Late-night salivary cortisol

The midnight salivary cortisol test can be done at home, as salivary cortisol remains stable at room temperature. The patient collects a saliva sample at midnight using a salivette and then brings it to the laboratory the next day. In healthy individuals the cortisol in both serum and saliva reaches a nadir after going to sleep. The natural circadian rhythm of cortisol is disrupted in Cushing's syndrome which leads to persistently raised cortisol levels even late at night. This test needs to be repeated at least twice.

False positive and false negative results

Immunoassays may increase the false positive rate [33], because of cross-reactivity with cortisone, which the salivary glands convert from cortisol via 11β-hydroxysteroid dehydrogenase type 2 [34]. Salivary cortisol increases with age, hypertension, and diabetes and patients with these conditions may therefore have false positive results [35].

FURTHER INVESTIGATIONS TO ESTABLISH THE CAUSE OF ENDOGENOUS HYPERCORTISOLAEMIA

Serum adrenocorticotrophic hormone measurement

Following a diagnosis of Cushing's syndrome a plasma ACTH level may be useful to distinguish between an ACTH-independent and ACTH-dependent cause. A low plasma ACTH concentration (< 10 pg/mL) is suggestive of an adrenal cause whereas a high ACTH

Table 3.4 Medical therapy options for Cushing's syndrome		
Drug and dose regime	**Mode of action**	**Side-effects**
Site of action: pituitary		
Pasireotide	Somatostatin analogue (binds to receptor subtypes 1, 2, 3 and 5)	GI symptoms, sinus bradycardia, cholelithiasis **Risk:** hyperglycaemia
Cabergoline	Dopamine receptor subtype 2 agonist	Dizziness, nausea, postural hypotension Possibility of valvular heart disease
Site of action: adrenal cortex		
Metyrapone	Inhibits 11β-hydroxylase	GI symptoms, rash, dizziness, ataxia, hirsutism, acne, oedema, hypertension and hypokalaemia
Ketoconazole	Inhibits several steroidogenic enzymes	GI symptoms, reversible increase in aspartate aminotransferase and alanine aminotransferase, rash, sedation **Risk:** severe hepatotoxicity, hypogonadism in men
Mitotane	Inhibits several steroidogenic enzymes	GI symptoms, neurological effects (dizziness, ataxia, vertigo, decreased memory, confusion), dyslipidaemia **Risk:** potential teratogen and can cause abortion
Etimodate	Inhibiting 11β-hydroxylase and cholesterol sidechain cleavage	Requires monitoring in intensive care unit
Site of action: glucocorticoid receptor		
Mifepristone	Glucocorticoid receptor antagonist	GI symptoms, hypoadrenalism, hypokalaemia, hypertension, irregular menses, endometrial hyperplasia, rash
GI, gastrointestinal.		

Adrenocorticotrophic hormone – lowering agents

Cabergoline is a dopamine agonist mainly used for treatment of prolactinomas for tumour shrinkage and reduction in prolactin secretion. Corticotroph adenomas may express dopamine receptors. About 35% of patients treated by high doses of carbergoline for Cushing's disease achieve significant reduction in cortisol levels, but only 30% sustain a long-term effect [51].

Pasireotide is a somatostatin agonist with a particular binding affinity for somatostatin receptor isoforms 1, 2, 3 and 5. Pasireotide is associated with a risk of inducing or worsening pre-existing hyperglycaemia. A double-blind randomised controlled trial showed a significant decrease in cortisol levels in participants with Cushing's disease [52], but the side effects make this a poor choice for patients with Cushing's syndrome.

Steroidogenesis inhibitors

Metyrapone is a pyridine derivative that blocks cortisol synthesis mainly through inhibition of 11β-hydroxylase. It achieves rapid and effective control of hypercortisolaemia in approximately 50% of patients with Cushing's syndrome [53].

Ketoconazole is an antifungal agent with steroidogenesis inhibitor effects linked to inhibition of cytochrome P450 enzymes [54]. It is reported to normalise cortisol levels in Cushing's disease in about 50% of cases. The major concern is hepatotoxicity and liver function tests must be monitored during treatment [55].

Mitotane is derived from the insecticide dichlorodiphenyldichloroethane (DDD) and inhibits side chain cleavage of cholesterol and also other cytochrome P450 enzymes (11α- and 18-hydroxylase). It has a direct toxic effect on the adrenal cortex. There is a 4-week delay to obtain maximal efficacy due to its accumulation in adipose tissue. Mitotane is primarily used in the treatment of advanced or inoperable adrenocortical carcinoma [56].

Etomidate is an intravenous anaesthetic agent. It inhibits cortisol synthesis by inhibiting CYP11B1 with 11β-hydroxylase activity, and cytochrome P450 at high concentrations. Etomidate is very effective in reducing cortisol levels, but is limited by the fact that it can only be used intravenously in an intensive care unit due to respiratory suppression and sedation [57]. It should therefore be reserved for severe states of hypercortisolaemia.

Glucocorticoid receptor antagonist

Mifepristone is currently the only available glucocorticoid receptor antagonist and is effective in controlling clinical signs of hypercortisolaemia. Drawbacks to its use include its mineralocorticoid mode of action resulting in a high risk of hypokalemia. In addition, there is no biochemical means to monitor the patient because cortisol levels remain unchanged or may rise during treatment [58].

Bilateral adrenalectomy

When hypercortisolaemia is severe or if pituitary surgery fails, then bilateral adrenalectomy can be considered as it resolves cortisol hypersecretion rapidly in the vast majority of cases, with a low risk of perioperative complications particularly when performed via the laparoscopic or retroperitoneoscopic approach [59,60]. In addition, bilateral adrenalectomy can be used as a primary treatment for pituitary Cushing's in selected cases. The major and expected side effect of bilateral adrenalectomy is adrenal insufficiency requiring lifelong replacement of glucocorticoid (hydrocortisone or prednisolone) and mineralocorticoid (fludrocortisone). Nelson's syndrome, which is pituitary tumour progression observed after adrenalectomy, is rare [61].

TREATMENT FOR ADRENAL CUSHING'S SYNDROME

Functional adrenal adenomas causing Cushing's syndrome should be treated with unilateral adrenalectomy [62]. A laparoscopic or retroperitoneoscopic approach is preferable as is it safe, effective and requires less time spent in hospital by the patient, when compared to open adrenalectomy. Glucocorticoid replacement is required post-operatively until the HPA axis recovers. After surgery adrenal cancer can be treated medically with steroidogenesis inhibitors and mitotane [63].

TREATMENT FOR ECTOPIC ACTH SECRETION

The histology of ectopic ACTH-secretory tumours and the presence of metastasis should guide management. Surgical resection should be the primary goal. If full resection is not possible then other options for biochemical and symptom control include tumour-specific chemothereapy, steroidogenesis inhibitors, mifepristone or bilateral adrenalectomy.

DISCUSSION AND CONCLUSIONS

The diagnosis of Cushing's syndrome is clinically challenging due to its nonspecific clinical features. Nontargeted screening results in large numbers of false positive diagnoses of Cushing's, and deciding who warrants screening is often the first challenge. Once a decision has been made to screen a patient, the second challenge lies in choosing the best combination of investigations to reduce the risk of false positive or false negative outcomes. When interpreting the tests one should not forget that many conditions cause physiological hypercortisolaemia, however distinguishing between Cushing's syndrome and pseudo Cushing's syndrome can be challenge. No test on its own has a 100% diagnostic accuracy and a combination of screening tests should therefore be used.

Once Cushing's syndrome has been diagnosed an ACTH level should be checked to determine whether it is due an ACTH-dependent source or ACTH-independent source (an adrenal source of autonomous cortisol). Surgery remains the mainstay of treatment for Cushing's disease and adrenal adenomas.

A combination of screening and diagnostic tests has enabled a step-by-step approach to establish the underlying cause of endogenous Cushing's syndrome. Surgical treatment remains the mainstay of management whilst the newer medical therapies in Cushing's syndrome are under further clinical evaluation. Due to the many pitfalls in the diagnosis and interpretation of the various tests, patient selection at the point of screening is the most crucial step in making an accurate diagnosis and preventing unnecessary invasive investigations and procedures. The involvement of the multidisciplinary team (surgeons, histopathologists, oncologists, radiologist and endocrinologist, chemical pathologists) throughout is essential for optimising patient care.

Key points for clinical practice

- Do not screen for Cushing's syndrome before a thorough clinical evaluation confirms your suspicion that the patient belongs to a group that warrants screening.
- Discriminatory clinical features of Cushing's syndrome include plethora, proximal muscle weakness, easy bruising and purple striae.
- Select your screening tests based on your patient's specifications to reduce risk of false positives or false negatives.
- Imaging should only be carried out after it has been established whether the underlying cause of Cushing's syndrome is ACTH dependent or ACTH independent due to the high prevalence of pituitary/adrenal incidentalomas.
- Involve the multidisciplinary team early to optimise patient care.

REFERENCES

1.   Lindsay JR, Nansel T, Baid S, Gumowski J, Nieman LK. Long-term impaired quality of life in Cushing's syndrome despite initial improvement after surgical remission. J Clin Endocrinol Metab 2006; 91:447–453.
2.   Wagenmakers MA, Netea-Maier RT, Prins JB, et al. Impaired quality of life in patients in long-term remission of Cushing's syndrome of both adrenal and pituitary origin: a remaining effect of long-standing hypercortisolism? Eur J Endocrinol 2012; 167:687–695.

3. Bolland MJ, Holdaway IM, Berkeley JE, et al. Mortality and morbidity in Cushing's syndrome in New Zealand. Clin Endocrinol (Oxf) 2011; 75:436–442.

4. van Haalen FM, Broersen LH, Jorgensen JO, Pereira AM, Dekkers OM. Management of endocrine disease: Mortality remains increased in Cushing's disease despite biochemical remission: a systematic review and meta-analysis. Eur J Endocrinol 2015; 172:R143–149.

5. Ntali G, Asimakopoulou A, Siamatras T, et al. Mortality in Cushing's syndrome: systematic analysis of a large series with prolonged follow-up. European journal of endocrinology / European Federation of Endocrine Societies 2013; 169:715–723.

6. Steffensen C, Bak AM, Rubeck KZ, Jorgensen JO. Epidemiology of Cushing's syndrome. Neuroendocrinol 2010; 92:1–5.

7. Valassi E, Santos A, Yaneva M, et al. The European Registry on Cushing's syndrome: 2-year experience. Baseline demographic and clinical characteristics. European journal of endocrinology/European Federation of Endocrine Societies 2011; 165:383–392.

8. Lindholm J, Juul S, Jorgensen JO, et al. Incidence and late prognosis of cushing's syndrome: a population-based study. The Journal of clinical endocrinology and metabolism 2001; 86:117–123.

9. Lacroix A, Feelders RA, Stratakis CA, Nieman LK. Cushing's syndrome. Lancet 2015; 386:913–927.

10. Daly AF, Tichomirowa MA, Beckers A. The epidemiology and genetics of pituitary adenomas. Best Prac Res Clin Endocrinol Metab 2009; 23:543–554.

11. Reincke M, Sbiera S, Hayakawa A, et al. Mutations in the deubiquitinase gene USP8 cause Cushing's disease. Nature genetics 2015; 47:31–38.

12. de Groot JW, Links TP, Themmen AP, et al. Aberrant expression of multiple hormone receptors in ACTH-independent macronodular adrenal hyperplasia causing Cushing's syndrome. Eur J Endocrinol 2010; 163:293–299.

13. Louiset E, Duparc C, Young J, et al. Intraadrenal corticotropin in bilateral macronodular adrenal hyperplasia. N Engl J Med 2013; 369:2115–2125.

14. Lacroix A, Bourdeau I, Lampron A, et al. Aberrant G-protein coupled receptor expression in relation to adrenocortical overfunction. Clin Endocrinol 2010; 73:1–15.

15. Assie G, Libe R, Espiard S, et al. ARMC5 mutations in macronodular adrenal hyperplasia with Cushing's syndrome. N Engl J Med 2013; 369:2105–2114.

16. Feelders RA, Pulgar SJ, Kempel A, Pereira AM. The burden of Cushing's disease: clinical and health-related quality of life aspects. Eur J Endocrinol 2012; 167:311–326.

17. Faggiano A, Pivonello R, Spiezia S, et al. Cardiovascular risk factors and common carotid artery caliber and stiffness in patients with Cushing's disease during active disease and 1 year after disease remission. J Clin Endocrinol Metab 2003; 88:2527–2533.

18. Rebellato A, Grillo A, Dassie F, et al. Ambulatory blood pressure monitoring-derived short-term blood pressure variability is increased in Cushing's syndrome. Endocrine 2014; 47:557–563.

19. Stuijver DJ, van Zaane B, Feelders RA, et al. Incidence of venous thromboembolism in patients with Cushing's syndrome: a multicenter cohort study. J ClinEndocrinol Metab 2011; 96:3525–3532.

20. Crespo I, Esther GM, Santos A, et al. Impaired decision-making and selective cortical frontal thinning in Cushing's syndrome. Clin Endocrinol (Oxf) 2014; 81:826–833.

21. Bourdeau I, Bard C, Forget H, et al. Cognitive function and cerebral assessment in patients who have Cushing's syndrome. Endocrinol Metab Clin North Am 2005; 34:357–369.

22. Bourdeau I, Bard C, Noel B, et al. Loss of brain volume in endogenous Cushing's syndrome and its reversibility after correction of hypercortisolism. J Clin Endocrinol Metab 2002; 87:1949–1954.

23. Hermus AR, Smals AG, Swinkels LM, et al. Bone mineral density and bone turnover before and after surgical cure of Cushing's syndrome. J Clin Endocrinol Metab 1995; 80:2859–2865.

24. Graversen D, Vestergaard P, Stochholm K, Gravholt CH, Jorgensen JO. Mortality in Cushing's syndrome: a systematic review and meta-analysis. Eur J Intern Med 2012; 23:278–282.

25. Dekkers OM, Horvath-Puho E, Jorgensen JO, , et al. Multisystem morbidity and mortality in Cushing's syndrome: a cohort study. J Clin Endocrinol Metab 2013; 98:2277–2284.

26. Clayton RN, Raskauskiene D, Reulen RC, Jones PW. Mortality and morbidity in Cushing's disease over 50 years in Stoke-on-Trent, UK: audit and meta-analysis of literature. J Clin Endocrinol Metab 2011; 96:632–642.

27. Ross EJ, Linch DC. Cushing's syndrome – killing disease: discriminatory value of signs and symptoms aiding early diagnosis. Lancet 1982; 2:646–649.

28. Nieman LK, Biller BM, Findling JW, Newell-Price J, Savage MO, Stewart PM, et al. The diagnosis of Cushing's syndrome: an Endocrine Society Clinical Practice Guideline. J Clin Endocrinol Metab 2008; 93:1526–1540.

29. Alwani RA, Schmit Jongbloed LW, et al. Differentiating between Cushing's disease and pseudo-Cushing's syndrome: comparison of four tests. Eur J Endocrinol 2014; 170:477–486.

30. Nickelsen T, Lissner W, Schoffling K. The dexamethasone suppression test and long-term contraceptive treatment: measurement of ACTH or salivary cortisol does not improve the reliability of the test. Exp Clin Endocrinol 1989; 94:275–280.

31. Chan KC, Lit LC, Law EL, et al. Diminished urinary free cortisol excretion in patients with moderate and severe renal impairment. Clin Chem 2004; 50:757–759.

32. Mericq MV, Cutler GB, Jr. High fluid intake increases urine free cortisol excretion in normal subjects. J Clin Endocrinol Metab 1998; 83:682–684.

33. Baid SK, Sinaii N, Wade M, Rubino D, Nieman LK. Radioimmunoassay and tandem mass spectrometry measurement of bedtime salivary cortisol levels: a comparison of assays to establish hypercortisolism. J Clin Endocrinol Metab 2007; 92:3102–3107.

34. Smith RE, Maguire JA, Stein-Oakley AN, et al. Localization of 11 beta-hydroxysteroid dehydrogenase type II in human epithelial tissues. J Clin Endocrinol Metab 1996; 81:3244–3248.

35. Liu H, Bravata DM, Cabaccan J, Raff H, Ryzen E. Elevated late-night salivary cortisol levels in elderly male type 2 diabetic veterans. Clin Endocrinol 2005; 63:642–649.

36. Aron DC, Raff H, Findling JW. Effectiveness versus efficacy: the limited value in clinical practice of high dose dexamethasone suppression testing in the differential diagnosis of adrenocorticotropin-dependent Cushing's syndrome. J Clin Endocrinol Metab 1997; 82:1780–1785.

37. Doppman JL, Chang R, Oldfield EH, et al. The hypoplastic inferior petrosal sinus: a potential source of false-negative results in petrosal sampling for Cushing's disease. J Clin Endocrinol Metab 1999; 84:533–540.

38. Findling JW, Kehoe ME, Raff H. Identification of patients with Cushing's disease with negative pituitary adrenocorticotropin gradients during inferior petrosal sinus sampling: prolactin as an index of pituitary venous effluent. J Clin Endocrinol Metab 2004; 89:6005–6009.

39. Booth GL, Redelmeier DA, Grosman H, et al. Improved diagnostic accuracy of inferior petrosal sinus sampling over imaging for localizing pituitary pathology in patients with Cushing's disease. J Clin Endocrinol Metab 1998; 83:2291–2295.

40. Doppman JL, Frank JA, Dwyer AJ, et al. Gadolinium DTPA enhanced MR imaging of ACTH-secreting microadenomas of the pituitary gland. J Comput Assist Tomogr 1988; 12:728–735.

41. Hall WA, Luciano MG, Doppman JL, Patronas NJ, Oldfield EH. Pituitary magnetic resonance imaging in normal human volunteers: occult adenomas in the general population. Ann Intern Med 1994; 120:817–820.

42. Nieman LK, Biller BM, Findling JW, et al. Treatment of Cushing's syndrome: An Endocrine Society Clinical Practice Guideline. J Clin Endocrinol Metab 2015; 100:2807–2831.

43. Hofmann BM, Hlavac M, Martinez R, Buchfelder M, Muller OA, Fahlbusch R. Long-term results after microsurgery for Cushing disease: experience with 426 primary operations over 35 years. J Neurosurg 2008; 108:9–18.

44. Hoybye C, Grenback E, Thoren M, et al. Transsphenoidal surgery in Cushing disease: 10 years of experience in 34 consecutive cases. J Neurosurg 2004; 100:634–638.

45. Shimon I, Ram Z, Cohen ZR, Hadani M. Transsphenoidal surgery for Cushing's disease: endocrinological follow-up monitoring of 82 patients. Neurosurg 2002; 51:57–61.

46. Atkinson AB, Kennedy A, Wiggam MI, McCance DR, Sheridan B. Long-term remission rates after pituitary surgery for Cushing's disease: the need for long-term surveillance. Clin Endocrinol 2005; 63:549–559.

47. Wagenmakers MA, Netea-Maier RT, van Lindert EJ. Repeated transsphenoidal pituitary surgery (TS) via the endoscopic technique: a good therapeutic option for recurrent or persistent Cushing's disease (CD). Clin Endocrinol 2009; 70:274–280.

48. Locatelli M, Vance ML, Laws ER. Clinical review: the strategy of immediate reoperation for transsphenoidal surgery for Cushing's disease. J Clin Endocrinol Metab 2005; 90:5478–5482.

49. Estrada J, Boronat M, Mielgo M, et al. The long-term outcome of pituitary irradiation after unsuccessful transsphenoidal surgery in Cushing's disease. N Engl J Med 1997; 336:172–177.

50. Castinetti F, Regis J, Dufour H, Brue T. Role of stereotactic radiosurgery in the management of pituitary adenomas. Nature reviews Endocrinol 2010; 6:214–223.

51. Godbout A, Manavela M, Danilowicz K, Beauregard H, Bruno OD, Lacroix A. Cabergoline monotherapy in the long-term treatment of Cushing's disease. Eur J Endocrinol 2010; 163:709–716.

52. Colao A, Petersenn S, Newell-Price J, et al. A 12-month phase 3 study of pasireotide in Cushing's disease. N Engl J Med 2012; 366:914–924.

53. Verhelst JA, Trainer PJ, Howlett TA, Perry L, Rees LH, Grossman AB, et al. Short and long-term responses to metyrapone in the medical management of 91 patients with Cushing's syndrome. Clin Endocrinol 1991; 35:169–178.
54. Fleseriu M, Petersenn S. Medical therapy for Cushing's disease: adrenal steroidogenesis inhibitors and glucocorticoid receptor blockers. Pituitary 2015; 18:245–252.
55. Castinetti F, Guignat L, Giraud P, et al. Ketoconazole in Cushing's disease: is it worth a try? J Clin Endocrinol Metab 2014; 99:1623–1630.
56. Terzolo M, Angeli A, Fassnacht M, et al. Adjuvant mitotane treatment for adrenocortical carcinoma. N Engl J Med 2007; 356:2372–2380.
57. Dabbagh A, Sa'adat N, Heidari Z. Etomidate infusion in the critical care setting for suppressing the acute phase of Cushing's syndrome. Anesth Analg 2009; 108:238–239.
58. Carmichael JD, Fleseriu M. Mifepristone: is there a place in the treatment of Cushing's disease? Endocrine 2013; 44:20–32.
59. Katznelson L. Bilateral adrenalectomy for Cushing's disease. Pituitary 2015; 18:269–273.
60. Constantinides VA, Christakis I, Touska P, Meeran K, Palazzo F. Retroperitoneoscopic or laparoscopic adrenalectomy? A single-centre UK experience. Surg Endosc 2013; 27:4147–4152.
61. Assie G, Bahurel H, Coste J, et al. Corticotroph tumor progression after adrenalectomy in Cushing's Disease: A reappraisal of Nelson's Syndrome. JClin Endocrinol Metab 2007; 92:172–179.
62. Nehs MA, Ruan DT. Minimally invasive adrenal surgery: an update. Current Opin Endocrinol Diabetes Obes 2011; 18:193–197.
63. Fassnacht M, Libe R, Kroiss M, Allolio B. Adrenocortical carcinoma: a clinician's update. Nat Rev Endocrinol 2011; 7:323–335.

Chapter 4

Tyrosine kinase inhibitors in the management of differentiated thyroid cancer

Jackie A Gilbert, Julian A Waung, Kate Newbold

INTRODUCTION

Thyroid cancer is the most common endocrine malignancy. Thyroid cancers are derived from two types of endocrine thyroid cells – follicular cells and parafollicular C cells. Follicular thyroid cell-derived tumours include papillary thyroid cancer (PTC), follicular thyroid cancer (FTC), poorly-differentiated thyroid cancer (PDTC) and anaplastic thyroid cancer (ATC). Collectively, PTC and FTC are called differentiated thyroid cancer (DTC) and constitute the majority of thyroid cancers.

The long-term prognosis of most DTC is favourable with a 10-year survival of 80–90% for middle-aged adults [1]. However, 5–20% of patients develop local or regional recurrence and 10–15% distant metastases. High-risk, recurrent and metastatic disease is managed with total thyroidectomy and radioiodine. However, radioactive iodine (RAI) is curative in less than half of patients with metastatic disease. In those who are not responsive to RAI, cytotoxic chemotherapy has been of limited benefit with considerable morbidity [2]; median survival is 3–4 years [3]. There has been significant progress in our understanding of the molecular pathogenesis of thyroid cancer [4]. This has enabled the development of targeted therapies that have become the new standard of care for progressive RAI-refractory DTC (RR-DTC). These targeted therapies, although effective, are associated with specific adverse effects that may limit tolerability. Therefore both patient selection and the decision of when to initiate treatment are critical to ensure the optimum balance between benefit and toxicity.

Jackie A Gilbert MB PhD FRCP, Department of Endocrinology, King's College Hospital, London, UK. Email: jackiegilbert@nhs.net (for correspondence).

Julian A Waung MB MRCP, Department of Endocrinology, Hammersmith Hospital, London, UK.

Kate Newbold MB ChB MRCP FRCR FRCPE, Thyroid Unit, Royal Marsden Hospital, London, UK.

SIGNALLING PATHWAYS AND MECHANISMS OF GENETIC ALTERATION IN DIFFERENTIATED THYROID CANCER

The molecular pathogenesis of the majority of DTC involves the dysregulation of the mitogen-activated protein kinase (MAPK) and phosphatidylinositol-3 kinase (PI3K)/AKT signalling pathways (**Figure 4.1**).

A comprehensive, multiplatform analysis from nearly 500 PTCs identified a *BRAF* gene mutation in more than 60% of tumours [5]. Of these, the majority were the T1799A point mutation of *BRAF* responsible for the BRAF-V600E oncoprotein that results in constitutive activation of this signalling pathway. *BRAF-V600E* mutation occurs in 45% of PTC [6]. *BRAF-V600E* mutations signal as a monomer and therefore are not responsive to the negative feedback from ERK to RAF, resulting in high MAPK-signalling (**Figure 4.1**).

RAS genes (*HRAS*, *KRAS*, and *NRAS*) encode G proteins that are dual activators of the MAPK and PI3K/AKT pathways. Point mutations are found in 40–50% of FTC and 10–20%

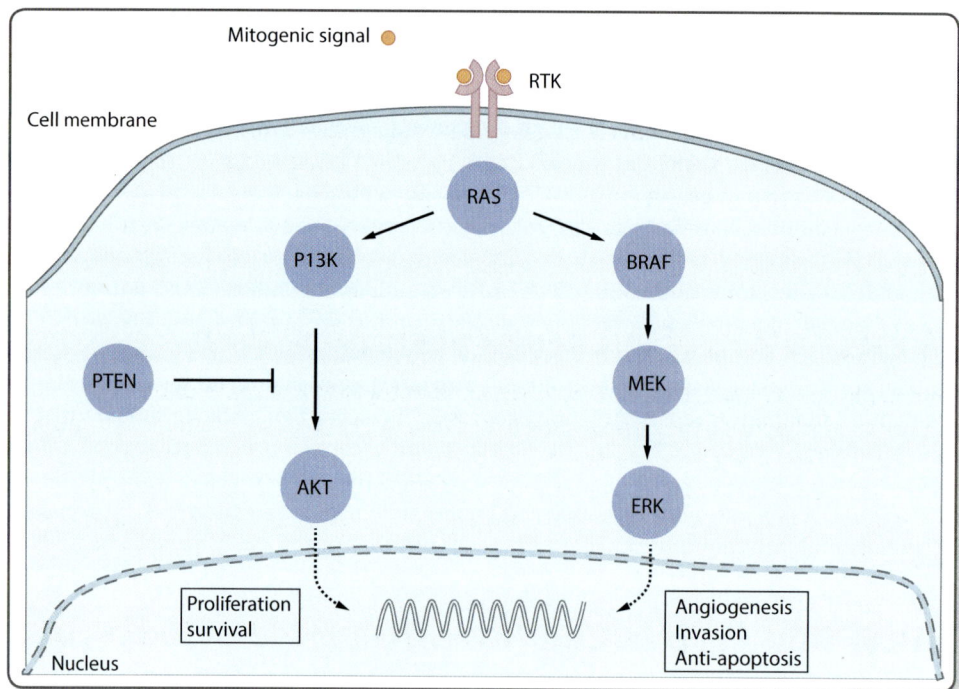

Figure 4.1 An extracellular mitogenic signal binds to receptor tyrosine kinase (RTK) on the surface of thyroid follicular cells, leading to dimerisation and phosphorylation of tyrosine residues in the cytoplasmic tail. This triggers downstream signalling of mitogen-activated protein kinase (MAPK) and phosphatidylinositol-3 kinase (PI3K) pathways through phosphorylation. Activated extracellular-signal-regulated kinase (ERK) and AKT migrate to the nucleus where they phosphorylate and activate various transcription factors that regulate cell survival and proliferation. Genetic alterations occur at various points of the pathway leading to constitutive activation of one or multiple pathways. Genetic translocation of RET with a partner gene can lead to ligand-independent dimerisation and constitutive tyrosine kinase activity of RET. Alternatively, copy number gain of RTK can drive tumourigenesis. Point mutations occur in *RAS* and most commonly RAF (*BRAF-V600E*). PTEN is a tumour-suppressor gene whose function can be lost through germline mutation (Cowden's syndrome) or epigenetic mechanism such as hypermethylation.

of PTC [8]. In contrast to *BRAF-V600E* mutations, tumours driven by *RAS* and receptor tyrosine kinase (RTK) fusions signal via RAF dimers that respond to ERK feedback, resulting in lower MAPK-signalling [5]. Therefore, *RAS* mutations lead to constitutive activation with a preference for the PI3K-AKT pathway.

The RET proto-oncogene encodes for a RTK. Activating point mutations lead to the development of medullary thyroid cancer. A chromosomal rearrangement resulting from genetic translocation of the 3′ tyrosine kinase portion of RET and the 5′ portion of a partner gene leads to the fusion oncoprotein RET-PTC. This results in ligand-independent dimerisation and constitutive tyrosine kinase activity of RET [4]. RET-PTC activates MAPK and PI3K-AKT pathways and occurs in classical PTC, follicular variant PTC (FVPTC) but also benign thyroid lesions [9]. The paired box 8 (*PAX8*) – peroxisome proliferator-activated receptor-γ (*PPARG*) fusion gene (*PAX8–PPARG*) is another prominent recombinant oncogene in thyroid cancer, occurring in up to 60% of FTC and FVPTC [4].

RTKs also contribute to tumourigenesis through copy number gain [10]. This mechanism of gene amplification is also seen in members of the PI3K-AKT pathway [4]. Aberrant gene methylation silences a gene when it occurs in its promoter region. This epigenetic mechanism of tumourigenesis occurs in BRAF-V600E mutation where tumour suppressor genes such as tissue inhibitor of metalloproteinase 3, SLC5A8, death-associated protein kinase 1 and retinoic acid receptor β are silenced [11]. Various genetic alterations to the PI3K-AKT pathway are associated with hypermethylation of phosphatase and tensin homolog (*PTEN*), a tumour suppressor gene. The resultant silencing of *PTEN* impairs its ability to modulate PI3K-AKT pathway activation and therefore creates a positive feedback loop [12]. Alternatively, germline loss of function mutations or deletions in the tumour suppressor gene *PTEN* underlie the 70-fold increase risk of DTC in Cowden's syndrome [13].

KINASE INHIBITORS – MECHANISM OF ACTION

Protein phosphorylation, regulated by kinases and phosphatases, is a common and important mechanism of post-translational modification to regulate function. The central role of kinase signalling in cancer tumour biology makes it a rational drug target. The constitutive kinase activity of cancer cells renders them exceptionally susceptible to inhibition whilst normal cells are able to tolerate such inhibition enabling the selective targeting of these agents [14].

MULTI-TARGETED KINASE INHIBITORS LICENSED FOR DTC

Sorafenib

Sorafenib is an oral kinase inhibitor of VEFG receptors 1, 2, 3; RET (including RET/PTC), RAF (including *BRAF-V600E*), and PDGFR-b. sorafenib is the most extensively studied drug for the treatment of RR-DTC with several phase 2 trials of heterogeneous design and inclusion criteria [17-21]. Favourable outcomes from these studies led to the randomised, double-blind, placebo-controlled, phase 3 DECISION study [22]. Patients with RAI-refractory, locally advanced or metastatic DTC (*n* = 417) that had progressed within the preceding 14 months were treated with 400 mg of sorafenib twice daily or placebo. The primary endpoint was progression-free survival (PFS) according to response evaluation criteria in solid tumors (RECIST) [23]. A significant improvement in PFS was observed in the sorafenib-treated subjects compared with placebo (10.8 and 5.8 months; HR 0.59, 95% CI 0.45–0.76; $p < 0.0001$). The partial response rate in sorafenib and placebo was 12.2% and 0.5% ($p < 0.0001$) whilst stable disease at 6 months was observed in 42% and 33% respectively. Of note, 71% of patients randomised to placebo crossed over to sorafenib treatment at the point of disease progression. An analysis of disease biomarkers showed that *BRAF* and *RAS* mutations were neither independently prognostic nor predictive of sorafenib benefit.

Adverse events occurred in 98.6% of patients taking sorafenib. The most frequent treatment-emergent events were hand-foot skin reactions (76%), diarrhoea (68%), alopecia (67%), rash or desquamation (50%) and hypertension (41%). Adverse events occurred in 87.6% of patients taking placebo suggesting that the disease itself was causing a significant number of symptoms. Although the sorafenib-related toxicities were mainly grade 1 or 2, dose interruption, reductions or withdrawals occurred in 66%, 64% and 18% of patients respectively. Based on the strength of this study, sorafenib has been approved by the US Food and Drug Administration (FDA) and the European Medicines Agency (EMA) for the treatment of progressive DTC. It is currently available in England through the National Cancer Drugs Fund.

Lenvatinib

Lenvatinib is an inhibitor of vascular endothelial growth factor receptor (VEGFR), fibroblast growth factor (FGF) receptor 1, 2 and 3, RET, KIT and PDGRF. In a double blind multicentre phase-3 study (SELECT), 392 patients with RAI-refractory progressive DTC were randomised to 24 mg of lenvatinib once a day or placebo in a 2:1 ratio [24]. A significant improvement in the primary endpoint, PFS according to RECIST, was observed with lenvatinib compared to placebo (18.3 versus 3.6 months; HR for progression or death 0.21; 99% CI 0.14–0.31; $p < 0.001$). The response rate was 64.8% in the lenvatinib group (4 complete responses and 165 partial responses) and 1.5% (2 partial responses) in the placebo group; (OR 28.87; 95% CI, 12.46–66.86; $p < 0.001$). Lenvatinib was equally efficacious for different tumour histological types and mutation status (*BRAF* or *RAS*).

Adverse events occurred in 97.3% of patients assigned lenvatinib, with 76% being grade 3 or higher. The most common adverse effects were hypertension (69%), diarrhoea (59%), fatigue (59%), nausea (41%) and anorexia (50%). The FDA and EMA have licensed lenvatinib for the treatment of RR-DTC. It is currently not funded in the UK.

ANALYSIS OF DECISION AND SELECT TRIALS

Both sorafenib and lenvatinib demonstrated clear efficacy compared to placebo for PFS. However, no study has been able to show a benefit in overall survival in patients with DTC treated with kinase inhibitor. Additionally, both sorafenib and lenvatinib demonstrated considerable toxicity, necessitating dose interruption, reduction or cessation of drugs in 66–82%, 64–68% and 14–19% respectively (**Table 4.1**). Diarrhoea, fatigue, anorexia and weight loss are common with both drugs. However, cutaneous reactions are more common with sorafenib. In comparison, hypertension and proteinuria, which have been observed as a class effect with VEGFR inhibitors, were more common with lenvatinib treatment.

There are no trials directly comparing sorafenib and levantinib, making it impossible to compare their efficacy. However, there are a few notable differences between the patients and outcomes in the DECISION and SELECT studies: SELECT had a higher proportion of patients with bone metastases (39.8% versus 27.5%) and patients treated previously with systemic therapy (25.3% versus 3.4%) compared to DECISION.

Table 4.1 Comparison of sorafenib and lenvatinib in phase III clinical trials*		
	Sorafenib	Lenvatinib
Demographics (%)		
Median age (years)	63	64
Male	50.2	47.9
ECOG 0-1	96.1	95
Histology (%)		
Papillary	57	50.6
Poorly differentiated	11.6	10.7
Follicular (non-Hurtle)	17.9	20.3
Hurtle cell	6.3	18.4
Metastases (%)		
Bone	27.5	39.8
Lung	86	86.9
One prior TKI (%)	3.4	25.3
Adverse events (%)		
Hypertension	41	69
Proteinuria	Not reported	32
Diarrhoea	68	59
Fatigue	50	59
Nausea	21	41
Appetite decrease	32	50
Weight loss	47	46
Hand-foot skin reaction	76	32
Alopecia	67	11
Rash or desquamation	50	16
Serum TSH increase	33	62
Effect of adverse effects on dosing		
Dose interruption	66	82
Dose reduction	64	68
Withdrawal	19	14
Mean dose (mg)	651	17
Mean dose as % starting dose	81	86

ECOG, Eastern Cooperative Oncology Group (ECOG) Performance Status; TKI, tyrosine kinase inhibitor.
*Adapted from Brose et al. [22] and Schlumberger et al. [25]

Patient selection for systemic therapy

Multikinase inhibitors have provided a treatment option for patients who have progressive RR-DTC, where previously there was no disease modifying treatment and patients were treated with best supportive care. To date these kinase inhibitors have proven to prolong PFS but have not been shown to reduce mortality and are associated with not insignificant

toxicity. Therefore, considerable judgement is required to determine when to start therapy and how to select patients who will benefit most. An expert panel has proposed a working definition and treatment algorithm: Patients with RR-DTC have metastatic disease that does not take up iodine or the disease progresses despite substantial uptake of RAI. Those who are likely to benefit from systemic therapy have a large tumour burden and progressive disease according to RECIST criteria [25].

MANAGEMENT OF SIDE EFFECTS

Although the rates of treatment emergent adverse events were high in both trials, physicians treating patients with these drugs have since gained experience in how to manage the side effects by initial close monitoring and early intervention, thereby permitting better dose intensity by avoiding dose reductions and interruptions.

Dermatological

The risk of severe, cutaneous reactions should be reduced through patient education, early monitoring and dose reduction or interruption of kinase inhibitors when they occur. Patients should have an evaluation of their skin and mucosal surface prior to commencing kinase inhibitors. Strict photoprotection through avoidance of sun exposure, protective clothing and UVA/UVB sunscreen with a sun protection factor of 30 or higher should be recommended. Products that dry the skin (e.g. soaps or alcohol-based or perfumed products) should be avoided. Finally, vigilance is required as *BRAF* inhibitors such as sorafenib are associated with the development of cutaneous squamous cell cancers and keratoacanthomas in up to 5% of treated patients [26].

Cardiovascular

Blood pressure should be recorded prior to commencing therapy. Early monitoring for hypertension is essential and it can usually be treated with angiotensin converting enzyme (ACE) inhibitors. Calcium channel antagonists and beta-blockers can be used as additional antihypertensives. A 12-lead ECG should be recorded prior to drug initiation. Patients should be monitored for QTc prolongation and interfering concomitant medications avoided. The risk of QTc prolongation is a particular concern with vandetanib (used to treat medullary thyroid cancer) compared to the lower risk with sorafenib and lenvatinib.

Gastrointestinal

Dietary modification with soft food and more frequent, smaller portions may improve mild nausea and vomiting. Metoclopramide, a dopamine D2 receptor antagonist may be used as an antiemetic. 5-HT$_3$ antagonists such as ondansetron should be avoided as they have the potential to prolong QTc. Diarrhoea can be treated with loperamide and mild opioids such as codeine. Prompt replacement of electrolytes is critical to reduce the risk of potential cardiotoxicity.

Thyroid-stimulating hormone suppression

Thyroid-stimulating hormone (TSH) suppression remains a treatment goal in patients with RR-DTC. Increased levothyroxine doses are frequently required upon commencing kinase inhibitor therapy to achieve the desired TSH < 0.1 mU/L. This is consistent with

the observation that 32% and 62% of patients had an elevated TSH in the DECISION and SELECT trials, respectively. This may be a direct effect of the kinase inhibitor or be related to malabsorption secondary to drug-induced diarrhoea. Patients should be instructed to take levothyroxine in the fasted state and separate from other medication, especially proton pump inhibitors. Serum TSH levels should be monitored regularly.

SELUMETINIB-ENHANCED RADIOACTIVE IODINE UPTAKE IN THYROID CANCER

Metastatic thyroid cancer that retains RAI avidity has a 10-year survival rate of 60%. By contrast, this falls to 10% in metastatic disease that is refractory to radioiodine. Previous efforts to re-differentiate thyroid cancer cells using retinoids [27] and lithium [28] were of limited clinical benefit. In mouse models of thyroid cancer, selective MAPK pathway antagonists increase membrane expression of the sodium iodide symporter and hence iodide uptake. Therefore, a study of 24 patients with RR-DTC investigated whether selective MAPK inhibition would enhance RAI sensitivity [29]. Recombinant-TSH stimulated iodine-124 PET scans were performed before and 4 weeks after therapy with selumetinib 75 mg twice daily, a MEK1 and MEK2 inhibitor. Selumetinib increased radioiodine uptake in 12 of the 20 patients, with 8 reaching the dosimetric threshold for radioiodine therapy. Of those treated, 5 had partial responses and 3 had stable disease, with all patients demonstrating a fall in serum thyroglobulin level. This study was an important proof of principle that MAPK inhibition can enhance radioiodine uptake. However, kinase inhibitors are not currently used in routine clinical practice as an adjuvant therapy to improve RAI responsiveness. This is the subject of ongoing clinical trials.

CONCLUSION

Increased understanding of the molecular pathogenesis of DTC has enabled the parallel development of kinase inhibitors. This rationally designed and efficacious class of drugs has become the standard of care for the minority of thyroid cancer patients with progressive, radioiodine refractory disease. Clinicians involved in the care of thyroid cancer patients are likely to encounter this class of drugs with increasing frequency in the future. These drugs should only be initiated by experienced specialists in order to effectively manage toxicities and thereby maximise the clinical benefit. Further work is needed to develop more selective inhibitors, combat drug resistance and minimise toxicity.

Key points for clinical practice

- Patients with progressive RR-DTC disease should be considered for multikinase inhibitor therapy.
- Multikinase inhibitors prolong PFS but have not been demonstrated to reduce mortality.
- Adverse effects may limit tolerability and therefore patient selection and timing of treatment initiation are extremely important.
- Multitargeted kinase inhibitors should only be initiated by clinicians experienced in their use.

REFERENCES

1.   Perros P, Boelaert K, Colley S, et al. Guidelines for the management of thyroid cancer. Clin Endocrinol (Oxf) 2014; 81 S1:1–122.
2.   Sherman SI. Cytotoxic chemotherapy for differentiated thyroid carcinoma. Clin Oncol (R Coll Radiol) 2010; 22:464–468.
3.   Durante C, Haddy N, Baudin E, et al. Long-term outcome of 444 patients with distant metastases from papillary and follicular thyroid carcinoma: benefits and limits of radioiodine therapy. J Clin Endocrinol Metab 2006; 91:2892–2899.
4.   Xing M. Molecular pathogenesis and mechanisms of thyroid cancer. Nat Rev Cancer 2013; 13:184–199.
5.   Cancer Genome Atlas Research Network. Integrated genomic characterization of papillary thyroid carcinoma. Cell 2014; 159:676–690.
6.   Xing M. BRAF mutation in thyroid cancer. Endocr Relat Cancer 2005; 12:245–262.
7.   Xing M, Westra WH, Tufano RP, et al. BRAF mutation predicts a poorer clinical prognosis for papillary thyroid cancer. J Clin Endocrinol Metab 2005; 90:6373–6379.
8.   Hsiao SJ, Nikiforov YE. Molecular approaches to thyroid cancer diagnosis. Endocr Relat Cancer 2014; 21:301–313.
9.   Marotta V, Guerra A, Sapio MR, Vitale M. RET/PTC rearrangement in benign and malignant thyroid diseases: a clinical standpoint. Eur J Endocrinol 2011; 165:499–507.
10. Liu Z, Hou P, Ji M, et al. Highly prevalent genetic alterations in receptor tyrosine kinases and phosphatidylinositol 3-kinase/AKT and mitogen-activated protein kinase pathways in anaplastic and follicular thyroid cancers. J Clin Endocrinol Metab 2008; 93:3106–3116.
11. Hu S, Liu D, Tufano RP, et al. Association of aberrant methylation of tumor suppressor genes with tumor aggressiveness and BRAF mutation in papillary thyroid cancer. Int J Cancer 2006; 119:2322–2329.
12. Hou P, Xing M. Association of PTEN gene methylation with genetic alterations in the phosphatidylinositol 3-kinase/AKT signaling pathway in thyroid tumors. Cancer 2008; 113:2440–2447.
13. Ngeow J, Mester J, Rybicki LA, et al. Incidence and clinical characteristics of thyroid cancer in prospective series of individuals with Cowden and Cowden-like syndrome characterized by germline PTEN, SDH, or KLLN alterations. J Clin Endocrinol Metab 2011; 96:2063–2071.
14. Zhang J, Yang PL, Gray NS. Targeting cancer with small molecule kinase inhibitors. Nat Rev Cancer 2009; 9:28–39.
15. O'Brien SG, Guilhot F, Larson RA, et al. Imatinib compared with interferon and low-dose cytarabine for newly diagnosed chronic-phase chronic myeloid leukemia. N Engl J Med 2003; 348:994–1004.
16. Gaumann AK, Kiefer F, Alfer J, et al. Receptor tyrosine kinase inhibitors: Are they real tumor killers? Int J Cancer 2016; 138:540–554.
17. Ahmed M, Barbachano Y, Riddell A, et al. Analysis of the efficacy and toxicity of sorafenib in thyroid cancer: a phase II study in a UK based population. Eur J Endocrinol 2011; 165:315–22.
18. Gupta-Abramson V, Troxel AB, Nellore A, et al. Phase II trial of sorafenib in advanced thyroid cancer. J Clin Oncol 2008; 26:4714–4719.
19. Hoftijzer H, Heemstra KA, Morreau H, et al. Beneficial effects of sorafenib on tumor progression, but not on radioiodine uptake, in patients with differentiated thyroid carcinoma. Eur J Endocrinol 2009; 161:923–931.
20. Kloos RT, Ringel MD, Knopp MV, et al. Phase II trial of sorafenib in metastatic thyroid cancer. J Clin Oncol 2009; 27:1675–1684.
21. Schneider TC, Abdulrahman RM, Corssmit EP, et al. Long-term analysis of the efficacy and tolerability of sorafenib in advanced radio-iodine refractory differentiated thyroid carcinoma: final results of a phase II trial. Eur J Endocrinol 2012; 167:643–650.
22. Brose MS, Nutting CM, Jarzab B, et al. Sorafenib in radioactive iodine-refractory, locally advanced or metastatic differentiated thyroid cancer: a randomised, double-blind, phase 3 trial. Lancet 2014; 384:319–328.
23. Eisenhauer EA, Therasse P, Bogaerts J, et al. New response evaluation criteria in solid tumours: revised RECIST guideline (version 1.1). Eur J Cancer 2009; 45:228–247.
24. Schlumberger M, Tahara M, Wirth LJ, et al. Lenvatinib versus placebo in radioiodine-refractory thyroid cancer. N Engl J Med 2015; 372:621–630.
25. Schlumberger M, Brose M, Elisei R, et al. Definition and management of radioactive iodine-refractory differentiated thyroid cancer. Lancet Diabetes Endocrinol 2014; 2:356–358.

26. Dubauskas Z, Kunishige J, Prieto VG, et al. Cutaneous squamous cell carcinoma and inflammation of actinic keratoses associated with sorafenib. Clin Genitourin Cancer 2009; 7:20–23.

27. Coelho SM, Corbo R, Buescu A, Carvalho DP, Vaisman M. Retinoic acid in patients with radioiodine non-responsive thyroid carcinoma. J Endocrinol Invest 2004; 27:334–339.

28. Liu YY, van der Pluijm G, Karperien M, et al. Lithium as adjuvant to radioiodine therapy in differentiated thyroid carcinoma: clinical and in vitro studies. Clin Endocrinol 2006; 64:617–624.

29. Ho AL, Grewal RK, Leboeuf R, et al. Selumetinib-enhanced radioiodine uptake in advanced thyroid cancer. N Engl J Med 2013; 368:623–632.

Chapter 5

Adrenal tumours

Paul C Dent, Fausto Palazzo

INTRODUCTION

The adrenal glands are situated in the retroperitoneum on the transpyloric plane approximately at the level of the first lumbar vertebra. The normal right adrenal gland is grossly triangular, moulded in part by its proximity with the liver, the right crus of the diaphragm and the inferior vena cava (IVC). The left gland is typically cresenteric. Each gland typically lies just superior and medial to the superior pole of the kidney. The arterial blood supply to the adrenal gland comes from branches of the inferior phrenic artery, the aorta and the ipsilateral renal artery. The venous drainage is through a vein direct to the IVC on the right and a vein draining into the renal vein and phrenic vein on the left.

Each adrenal gland is encased in a connective tissue pseudocapsule, and the distinct embryological origins of the adrenal cortex and medulla reflect two functionally distinct regions. The outer adrenal cortex is of mesodermal origin and an inner adrenal medulla derives from the neural crest and is therefore ectodermal in origin. The adrenal cortex represents approximately 85% of the gland and is subdivided into three zones from superficial to deep: the zona glomerulosa with columnar cells containing little cytoplasm and relatively large nuclei that produce mineralocorticoids; the zona fasiculata with polyhedral cells producing glucocorticoids; and the zona reticularis with rounded branching cords of cells that produce sex hormones. The adrenal medulla is populated with large columnar-shaped chromaffin cells with polymorphic nuclei and produces catecholamines including noradrenaline and adrenaline from a tyrosine substrate.

INCIDENTAL ADRENAL TUMOURS – 'THE ADRENAL INCIDENTALOMA'

Adrenal nodules were previously rarely detected and found only at post mortem or in patients with syndromes related to hormonal excess. However, the increasing use of cross sectional imaging over the last 3 decades has led to the detection of asymptomatic adrenal growths. The term 'adrenal incidentoma' has been adopted to describe radiologically detected adrenal tumours greater than 1 cm identified when adrenal disease was not the primary indication for the imaging performed. Approximately 4% of abdominal computed tomographic (CT) scans have identified adrenal incidentalomas [1] and the prevalence

Paul C Dent BMedSc (Hons) MB ChB (Hons) PhD FRCS (Gen), General and Endocrine Surgery, Hammersmith Hospital, London, UK. Email: pcdent@doctors.org.uk (for correspondence).

Fausto Palazzo MS FRCS (Gen), Department of Thyroid and Endocrine Surgery, Hammersmith Hospital, London, UK.

increases with age. Less than 1% are found in the third decade to over 7% in the eighth decade [2] but this is in part a product of detection bias given that cross-sectional imaging use increases with age [2,3].

Adrenal tumours may be classified on the basis of their anatomy as unilateral or bilateral, benign or malignant or according to their hyper-functionality potentially causing a syndrome that will vary according to the hormonal excess.

Most incidentalomas are benign non-functioning adenomas but other causes include benign connective tissue tumours (such as myelolipomas), haemorrhage into adrenal nodules, cortical cysts, haemangiomata, ganglioneuromas, lymphangiomas and congenital hyperplasia.

However, up to 15% of incidentalomas are hyperfunctional [4] including up to 10% that manifest catecholamine excess consistent with a phaeochromocytoma which can in many cases be completely asymptomatic [2,4,5]. Whilst the incidence of adrenal cancer of 0.7–2 cases per million per annum [6] makes a primary adrenocortical carcinoma rare, metastatic disease from an undiagnosed primary malignancy may be the cause of up to 2.5% of adrenal incidentalomas [7]. If the imaging is performed in a patient with a known malignancy the risk of the adrenal tumour representing metastatic spread climbs briskly to as high as 50% [8]. The most frequent malignancies that spread to the adrenal gland are lung, renal cell carcinoma and malignant melanoma but secondaries from breast and colorectal cancer may also occur [9].

The high incidence of incidental adrenal tumours contrasts with the low incidence of adrenocortical carcinoma (ACC) and asymptomatic adrenal hypersecretion and therefore requires rigorous clinical management protocols to identify clinically significant disease without exposing the patient to unnecessary surgery and further imaging with their associated risks and costs [5].

DIAGNOSIS

When an adrenal tumour is detected on imaging a complete clinical assessment is required to exclude symptoms or signs of hormonal hypersecretion such as atypical obesity, hypertension, diabetes, osteoporosis, virilisation or feminisation. A detailed history to exclude an underlying malignancy is required. Equally a thorough family history may unveil endocrinological syndromes especially but not exclusively in younger patients.

Even in normotensive asymptomatic patients, biochemical tests should be undertaken to exclude a functioning adrenal tumour.

Cushing's syndrome

Up to 20% of all functional adrenal adenomata hyper-secrete cortisol independent of circulating ACTH levels [4,5]. Patients with excess cortisol may report fatigue, proximal muscle wasting, increase in weight with central obesity, increased tendency to bruise, virilisation, new onset hypertension and glucose intolerance to frank diabetes. Biochemically, Cushing's syndrome may be diagnosed by high serum cortisol with a suppressed ACTH and a loss of the diurnal rhythm of plasma cortisol. The serum cortisol also fails to suppress appropriately on the administration of dexamethasone in the context of an overnight or low-dose dexamethasone suppression test. More recently, late night salivary cortisol testing has been shown to be a highly sensitive and specific screening test for Cushing's syndrome [10]. Many patients may over-secrete cortisol and have escaped the normal pituitary-adrenal cortex feedback mechanisms but insufficiently to have the clinical features of Cushing's syndrome. The concept of subclinical Cushing's syndrome was first described in 1973 by Beierwaltes and colleagues and has now been better defined biochemically [11,12]. The natural history of subclinical Cushing's on the skeleton, glucose metabolism and hypertension and therefore the optimal treatment approach remains the subject of debate [13]. Patients with SCCS who have undergone unilateral adrenalectomy have improved bone mineral density, suggesting that there is a long-term impact for these patients [14-16]. Similarly, a recent paper from Di Dalmazi and colleagues has suggested that patients with SCCS have an increased cardiovascular risk and an increased mortality rate compared to those with a non-secretory incidentaloma, although this paper is not without its critics [17]. However, the progression from SCCS to overt Cushing's syndrome is unpredictable and may only occur only in up to 12% of patients [18] with some studies suggesting spontaneous normalisation of endocrine function in up to 50% of cases [13,19]. The risk of developing cortisol oversecretion is greatest in patients with incidentalomas over 3 cm and studies are required to establish the role of surgery in selected cases of subclinical Cushing's syndrome [14]. Any patient undergoing surgery for an adrenal tumour should be assessed for hypercortisolism since post-operative steroid may be temporarily required to avoid the risk of an Addisonian crisis.

Conn's syndrome (primary hyperaldosteronism)

Conn's syndrome in its classic form is characterised by hypokalaemic hypertension. In cases where it is caused by a unilateral adrenal nodule these tend to be small, therefore Conn's syndrome is an uncommon diagnosis for an adrenal incidentaloma. Primary hyperaldosteronism is most commonly characterised by asymptomatic hypertension with or without hypokalaemia on biochemistry. The diagnosis is biochemical and based primarily on a screening protocol [20,21]. Primary hyperaldosteronism is biochemically characterised by a raised plasma aldosterone in the context of a suppressed renin activity level which distinguishes it from secondary hyperaldosteronism which has an extra-adrenal cause and is associated with an unsuppressed renin activity level. Numerous anti-hypertensive medications can affect the renin-angiotensin-aldosterone axis (aldosterone antagonists, beta-blockers and angiotensin-converting enzyme inhibitors) so these need to be discontinued prior to confirmatory tests including the saline suppression test although some controversy surrounds the value of some of the other tests such as the fludrocortisone suppression test [20,22,23]. Only half of patients with Conn's syndrome are hypokalaemic, but when present these patients require potassium supplements [4,20].

Dehydroepiandrostenedione sulphate and sex steroid hormone excess

Adrenal tumours associated with androgenising and feminising hormonal excess are considere to be primary malignancies until proven otherwise. Serum dehydroepiandrostenedione-sulphate (DHEA-S) may represent a marker in these circumstances [20,24]. However, there is a step-wise decrease in relation to age in normal subjects with wide variations between patients, bringing the overall utility of this test as an absolute measure into question [20,25].

Phaeochromacytoma

Up to 10% of incidentalomas are phaeochromocytomas [2,4] but the clinical presentation can be extremely varied. Presentations range from entirely asymptomatic to hypotensive collapse due to tumour infarction following a prolonged period of hypertension. However, the classic description is that of episodic severe hypertension characterised by headaches, sweating, tachycardia and marked pallor. Exclusion of phaeochromocytoma in all adrenal incidentalomas is therefore mandatory. The traditional urinary vanilmandelic acid (VMA) estimation has been surpassed by a 24-hour urine metanephrine and normetanephine estimation, which is both more sensitive and specific than VMA. Plasma-fractionated metanephrines and normetanephrines can also be used but are not universally available, are more expensive and require the patient to be supine for 20 minutes prior to phlebotomy. There is no consensus regarding the method of biochemical diagnosis and it is likely that availability, local guidelines and to an extent patient suitability will continue to determine the chosen method [26-28]. While 75% of phaeochromocytomas are sporadic in nature, the identification of syndromic forms justifies genetic screening particularly in patients under 50 years of age. Associated syndromes include multiple endocrine neoplasia type 2 caused by mutation in the *RET* gene, the *VHL* gene (von Hipple–Lindau disease), the neurofibromatosis-1 gene (*NF1*) or succinate dehydrogenase deficiency (SDH) mutations of which *SDHD* and *SDHB* are the most frequently encountered, especially in extra adrenal phaeochromocytomas.

Adrenocortical carcinoma

In the absence of local invasion or metastases, the diagnosis of ACC is histological. Up to 60% of ACC patients present with clinical features of hormone excess: Cushing's syndrome, mixed Cushing's and virilisation syndromes, hyperaldosteronism and virilisation, or virilisation alone. Patients with non-functioning ACC are identified by an incidental finding on abdominal imaging or less commonly by tumour enlargement causing abdominal symptoms [29-32].

ACC are mostly sporadic, however some occur as a component of hereditary cancer syndromes (see **Table 5.1**). Mutations on the *TP53* gene on chromosome 17 and also on several genes on chromosome 11 (*p15* and *q*) have also been implicated in sporadic ACC. In addition, genome studies of patients with ACC have identified somatic mutations in the beta-catenin pathway mediated by the *CTNNB1* gene as an independent predictor of less

Table 5.1 Hereditary syndromes associated with adrenocortical carcinoma		
Syndrome	Associated conditions	Chromosomal defect
Li–Fraumeni syndrome	Breast cancer, soft tissue and bone sarcoma, brain tumours and ACC	Inactivating mutations of the *TP53* tumour suppressor gene on chromosome 17p
Beckwith–Wiedemann syndrome	Wilms' tumour, neuroblastoma, hepatoblastoma, and ACC	Abnormalities in 11p15
Multiple endocrine neoplasia type 1	Parathyroid, pituitary and pancreatic neuroendocrine tumours and adrenal adenomas, as well as carcinomas	Inactivating mutations of the *MEN1* gene on chromosome 11q
SBLA syndrome	Sarcoma, breast and lung cancer, ACC, and other tumours	No chromosome defect identified

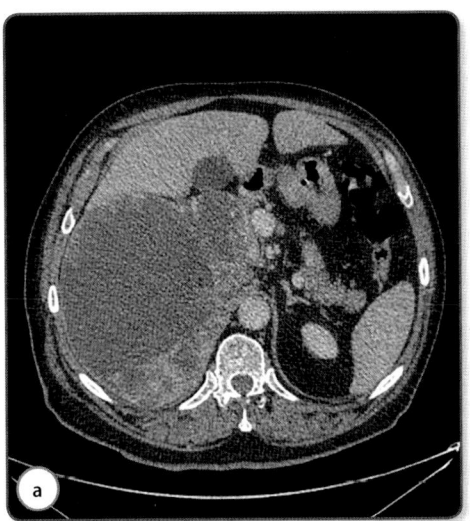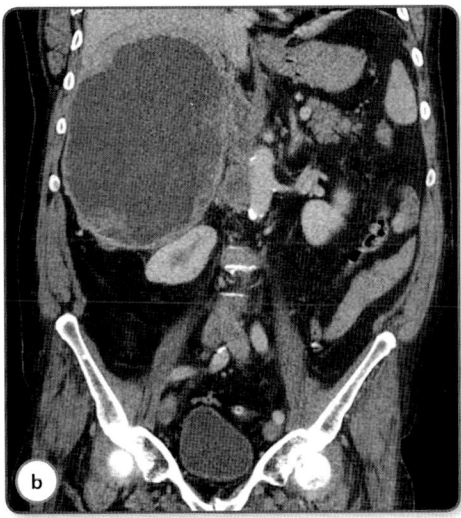

Figure 5.1 (a) Transaxial CT demonstrating an enlarged right adrenal gland with heterogenity and internal necrosis. (b) Coronal view of the same patient.

favourable disease-free and overall survival in patients following resection of ACC.

ACC are typically larger in size than benign adrenal cortex tumours and indeed the risk of ACC increases with size with 4 cm representing the point at which cancer risk begins to climb briskly (sensitivity, 97%; specificity, 52%), and 6 cm representing the point at which malignancy is an even more marked consideration (sensitivity, 91%; specificity, 80%). The risk of malignancy is however not exclusively size related, with the importance of radiological characteristics, biochemical profile and the age of the patient all relevant [33,34]. These form the basis of the recommendations of the British Association of Endocrine and Thyroid Surgeons (BAETS) [35]. There is of course concern that ACC start small, but counter intuitively several reports do not demonstrate that early detection of ACC improves survival [16]. Morphological features on imaging that are of concern include heterogeneity, internal haemorrhage or necrosis, irregular borders, and a high-contrast uptake with no washout phase (see **Figures 5.1**) [32]. MRI is comparable to CT scanning in its ability to identify ACC with a sensitivity of up to 89% and a specificity of up to 99% at distinguishing benign versus malignant masses [36,37]. Malignancy may be suggested by a hypointense signal on T1-weighted images and a hyperintense signal on T2-weighted images being representative of an increased fluid content [31]. PET scanning (see below) also has an increasing role when ACC is suspected.

ADVANCES IN RADIOLOGICAL ASSESSMENT OF ADRENAL TUMOURS

The most common modality for the assessment of the adrenal gland is computed tomography which may allow an initial malignancy risk assessment. Haemorrhage, cortical cysts, myelolipoma and benign adenomata have characteristic features on CT that allow immediate differentiation from malignant tumours and phaeochromocytoma in most cases.

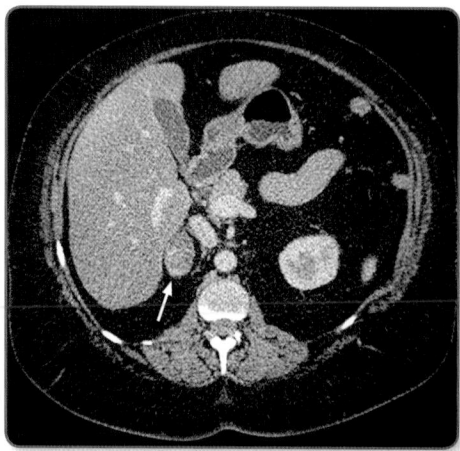

Figure 5.2 Right adrenal incidentaloma proved to be an ACTH-independent cortisol-secreting adenoma.

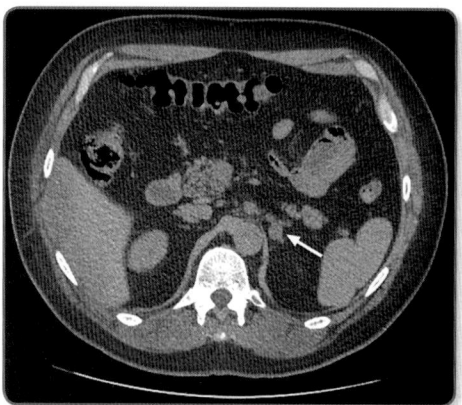

Figure 5.3 A small left adrenal adenoma. Functional studies demonstrated this to be an aldosterone secreting tumour.

Benign adenomata tend to have attenuation values below 10 Hounsfield units on non-contrast CT scans due to the relatively high intracellular lipid content (see **Figure 5.2**). Some benign adrenal lesions are not lipid rich and therefore may be confirmed by comparing scans immediately following intravenous contrast administration and then during a washout phase. Benign tumours have a tendency to show increased immediate enhancement (80–90 HU) and then washout on repeat scan (30–40 HU) [5,38,39].

Whilst adrenal protocol CT scanning is considered mandatory in surgical planning in Conn's syndrome, it does not reliably predict the side of aldosterone hypersecretion. This is due to the small size of these tumours (see **Figure 5.3**) and the frequent coexistence, especially in the older patient of a not entirely normal contralateral gland [20,21]. The current gold standard is adrenal vein sampling that allows the confirmation of the lateralisation of the disease and allows the identification of bilateral adrenal hyperaldosteronism that is treated with medication alone [40,41]. The objective is to assess the aldosterone/cortisol ratio in each of the adrenal veins, with a 3:1 gradient being diagnostic [21]. While adrenal vein sampling is the gold standard to lateralise disease prior to surgery, it can be technically demanding, unsuccessful or inconclusive. In expert hands however this is a very reliable test with minimal

management has similarly developed but there remains an unresolved challenge between surveillance and early surgery for those incidentalomas that are in the grey area for diagnostic criteria.

Key points for clinical practice

- There is a 4% incidence of adrenal incidentalomas in abdominal cross-sectional imaging.
- 15% are biochemically functional and may require further medical or surgical management.
- Phaeochromocytoma must be excluded before biopsy or surgery to prevent adrenal crisis. Identification of a phaeochromocytoma will require careful pre-operative planning and management.
- Discussion at a multi-disciplinary meeting with an adrenal surgeon, radiologist and endocrinologist will help both medical and/or surgical management planning, and long-term follow up.

REFERENCES

1. Bovio S, Cataldi A, Reimondo G, et al. Prevalence of adrenal incidentaloma in a contemporary computerized tomography series. J Endocrinol Invest 2006; 29:298.
2. Young WF Jr. Clinical practice. The incidentally discovered adrenal mass. N Engl J Med 2007; 356:601.
3. Terzolo M, Stigliano A, Chiodini I, et al. AME position statement on adrenal incidentaloma. Eur J Endocrinol 2011; 164:851.
4. Mantero F, Terzolo M, Arnaldi G, et al. A survey on adrenal incidentaloma in Italy. Study Group on Adrenal Tumors of the Italian Society of Endocrinology. J Clin Endocrinol Metab 2000; 85:637.
5. Reincke M. Subclinical Cushing's syndrome. Endocrinol Metab Clin North Am 2010; 29:43–56.
6. Kebebew E, Reiff E, Duh QY, et al. Extent of disease at presentation and outcome for adrenocortical carcinoma: have we made progress? World J Surg 2006; 30:872–878.
7. Cawood TJ, Hunt PJ, O'Shea D, et al. Recommended evaluation of adrenal incidentalomas is costly, has high false-positive rates and confers a risk of fatal cancer that is similar to the risk of the adrenal lesion becoming malignant; time for a rethink? Eur J Endocrinol 2009; 161:513.
8. Lenert JT, Barnett CC Jr, Kudelka AP, et al. Evaluation and surgical resection of adrenal masses in patients with a history of extra-adrenal malignancy. Surgery 2001; 130:1060–1067.
9. Hess KR, Varadhachary GR, Taylor SH, et al. Metastatic patterns in adenocarcinoma. Cancer 2006; 106:1624–1633.
10. Raff H. Cushing syndrome: update on testing. Endocrinol Metab Clin N Am 2015; 44:43–50.
11. Beierwaltes WH, Sturman MF, Ryo U, et al. Imaging functional nodules of the adrenal glands with 131-I-19-iodocholesterol. J Nucl Med 1974; 15:246–251.
12. Starker LF, Kunstman JW, Carling T. Subclinical Cushing syndrome: a review. Surg Clin North Am 2014; 94:657–668.
13. Rossi R, Tauchmanova L, Luciano A et al. Subclinical Cushing's syndrome in patients with adrenal incidentaloma: clinical and biochemical features. J Clin Endocrinol Metab 2000; 85:1440–1448.
14. Barzon L, Scaroni C, Sonino N, et al. Risk factors and long-term follow-up of adrenal incidentalomas. J Clin Endocrinol Metab 1999; 84:520–526.
15. Torlontano M, Chiodini I, Pileri M, et al. Altered bone mass and turnover in female patients with adrenal incidentaloma: the effect of subclinical hypercortisolism. J Clin Endocrinol Metab 1999; 84:2381–2385.
16. Toniato A, Merante-Boschin I, Opocher G, et al. Surgical versus conservative management for subclinical Cushing syndrome in adrenal incidentalomas: a prospective randomized study. Ann Surg 2009; 249:388–391.
17. Di Dalmazi G, Vicennati V, Garelli S, et al. Cardiovascular events and mortality in patients with adrenal incidentalomas that are either non-secreting or associated with intermediate phenotype or subclinical Cushing's syndrome: a 15-year retrospective study. Lancet Diabetes Endocrinol 2014; 2:396–405.

18. Barzon L, Fallo F, Sonino N, et al. Development of overt Cushing's syndrome in patients with adrenal incidentaloma. Eur J Endocrinol 2004; 146:61–66.
19. Terzolo M, Osella G, Alì A, et al. Subclinical Cushing's syndrome in adrenal incidentaloma. Clin Endocrinol 1998; 48:89–97.
20. Harvey AM. Hyperaldosteronism: diagnosis, lateralization, and treatment. Surg Clin North Am 2014; 94:643–656.
21. Funder JW, Carey RM, Fardella C, et al. Case detection, diagnosis, and treatment of patients with primary aldosteronism: an Endocrine Society clinical practice guideline. J Clin Endocrinol Metab 2008; 93:3266–3281.
22. Nanba K, Tamanaha T, Nakao K, et al. Confirmatory testing in primary aldosteronism. J Clin Endocrinol Metab 2012; 97:1688–1694.
23. Salva M, Cicala MV, Mantero F. Primary aldosteronism: the role of confirmatory tests. Horm Metab Res 2012; 44:177–180.
24. Allolio B, Fassnacht M. Clinical review: Adrenocortical carcinoma: clinical update. J Clin Endocrinol Metab 2006; 91:2027–37.
25. Orentreich N, Brind JL, Rizer RL, et al. Age changes and sex differences in serum dehydroepiandrosterone sulfate concentrations throughout adulthood. J Clin Endocrinol Metab 1984; 59:551-5.
26. Lenders JW, Pacak K, Walther MM, et al. Biochemical diagnosis of pheochromocytoma: which test is best? SOJAMA 2002; 287:1427.
27. Sawka AM, Jaeschke R, Singh RJ, et al. A comparison of biochemical tests for pheochromocytoma: measurement of fractionated plasma metanephrines compared with the combination of 24-hour urinary metanephrines and catecholamines. SOJ Clin Endocrinol Metab 2003;88:553.
28. Pacak K, Eisenhofer G, Ahlman H, et al. Pheochromocytoma: recommendations for clinical practice from the First International Symposium. October 2005. Nat Clin Pract Endocrinol Metab 2007; 3:92–102.
29. Aspinall SR, Imisairi AH, Bliss RD, et al. How is adrenocortical cancer being managed in the UK? Ann R Coll Surg Engl 2009; 91:489–93.
30. Else T, Kim AC, Sabolch A, et al. Adrenocortical carcinoma. Endocr Rev 2014; 35:282–326.
31. Libé R. Adrenocortical carcinoma (ACC): diagnosis, prognosis, and treatment. Front Cell Dev Biol 2015; 3:45.
32. Chagpar R, Siperstein AE, Berber, E. Adrenocortical cancer update. Surgical Clinics of North America 2014; 94: 669–687.
33. Sturgeon C, Shen WT, Clark OH et al. Risk assessment in 457 adrenal cortical carcinomas: how much does tumor size predict the likelihood of malignancy? J Am Coll Surg 2006; 202:423–430.
34. Blake MA, Holalkere NS, Boland GW. Imaging techniques for adrenal lesion characterization. Radiol Clin North Am 2008; 46:65–78.
35. The British Association of Endocrine and Thyroid Surgeons. Guidelines for the surgical management of endocrine disease and training requirements for endocrine surgery. London: The British Association of Endocrine and Thyroid Surgeons, 2003.
36. Honigschnabl S, Gallo S, Niederle B, et al. How accurate is MR imaging in characterisation of adrenal masses: update of a long-term study. Eur J Radiol 2002; 41:113–122.
37. Young WF Jr. Conventional imaging in adrenocortical carcinoma: update and perspectives. Horm Cancer 2011; 2:341–347.
38. Boland GW, Blake MA, Hahn PF, et al. Incidental adrenal lesions: principles, techniques, and algorithms for imaging characterization. Radiology 2008; 249:756–75.
39. Grumbach MM, Biller BM, Braunstein GD, et al. Management of the clinically inapparent adrenal mass ('incidentaloma'). Ann Intern Med 2003;138:424–429.
40. Young WF, Stanson AW, Thompson GB, et al. Role for adrenal venous sampling in primary aldosteronism. Surgery 2004; 136:1227–1235.
41. Zarnegar R, Bloom AI, Lee J, et al. Is adrenal venous sampling necessary in all patients with hyperaldosteronism before adrenalectomy? J Vasc Interv Radiol 2008; 19:66–71.
42. Burton T, Mackenzie I, Balan K, et al. Evaluation of the sensitivity and specificity of (11)C-metomidate positron emission tomography (PET)-CT for lateralizing aldosterone secretion by Conn's adenomas. J Clin Endocrinol Metab. 2012; 97:100–109.
43. Powlson A, Gurnell M, Brown M. Nuclear imaging in the diagnosis of primary aldosteronism. Curr Opin Endocrinol Diabetes Obes. 2015 ;22:150–156.
44. Hahner S, Stuermer A, Kreissl M, et al. [123 I]Iodometomidate for molecular imaging of adrenocortical cytochrome P450 family 11B enzymes. J Clin Endocrinol Metab 2008; 93:2358–2365.

45. Kreissl MC, Schirbel A, Fassnacht M, et al. [123I]Iodometomidate imaging in adrenocortical carcinoma. J Clin Endocrinol Metab 2013; 98:2755–2764.
46. Mukherjee JJ, Peppercorn, PD, Reznek, RH, et al. Pheochromocytoma: effect of nonionic contrast medium in CT on circulating catecholamine levels. Radiology 1997; 202:227–231.
47. Ilias I, Pacak K. Current approaches and recommended algorithm for the diagnostic localization of pheochromocytoma. J Clin Endocrinol Metab 2004; 89:479–491.
48. Ilias, I, Meristoudis G, Notopoulos A. A probabilistic assessment of the diagnosis of paraganglioma/pheochromocytoma based on clinical criteria and biochemical/imaging findings. Hell J Nucl Med 2015; 18:63–65.
49. Taieb D, Timmers HJ, Hindie E, et al. EANM 2012 guidelines for radionuclide imaging of phaeochromocytoma and paraganglioma. Eur J Nucl Med Mol Imaging 2012; 39:1977–1995.
50. Lenders JW, Duh OY, Eisenhofer G, et al Pheochromocytoma and paraganglioma: an endocrine society clinical practice guideline. J Clin Endocrinol Metab 2014; 99:1915–1942.
51. Castinetti F, Kroiss A, Kumar R, et al. 15 years of paraganglioma: Imaging and imaging-based treatment of pheochromocytoma and paraganglioma. Endocr Relat Cancer 2015; 22:T135–45.
52. Maurice JB, Troke R, Win Z, et al. A comparison of the performance of ^{68}Ga-DOTATATE PET/CT and ^{123}I-MIBG SPECT in the diagnosis and follow-up of phaeochromocytoma and paraganglioma. Eur J Nucl Med Mol Imaging 2012; 39:1266–1270.
53. Tan TH, Hussein Z, Saad ΓΓ, et al. Diagnostic performance of (68)Ga-DOTATATE PET/CT, (18)F-FDG PET/CT and (131)I-MIBG Scintigraphy in mapping metastatic pheochromocytoma and paraganglioma. Nucl Med Mol Imaging 2015; 49:143–151.
54. Angelousi A, Kassi E, Zografos G, et al. Metastatic pheochromocytoma and paraganglioma. Eur J Clin Invest 2015; 45:986–997.
55. Mojtahedi A, Thamake S, Tworowska I, et al. The value of 68Ga-DOTATATE PET/CT in diagnosis and management of neuroendocrine tumors compared to current FDA approved imaging modalities: a review of literature. Am J Nucl Med Mol Imaging 2014; 4:426–434.
56. Cistaro A, Niccoli Asabella A, Coppolino P, et al. Diagnostic and prognostic value of 18F-FDG PET/CT in comparison with morphological imaging in primary adrenal gland malignancies - a multicenter experience. Hell J Nucl Med 2015; 18:97–102.
57. Kim JY, Kim SH, Lee HJ, et al. Utilisation of combined 18F-FDG PET/CT scan for differential diagnosis between benign and malignant adrenal enlargement. Br J Radiol 2013; 86:20130190.
58. Groussin L, Bonardel G, Silvera S, et al. 18F-Fluorodeoxyglucose positron emission tomography for the diagnosis of adrenocortical tumors: a prospective study in 77 operated patients. J Clin Endocrinol Metab 2009; 94:1713–22.
59. Yankaskas BC, Staab EV, Craven MB, et al. Delayed complications from fine-needle biopsies of solid masses of the abdomen. Invest Radiol 1986; 21:325–8.
60. Habscheid W, Pfeiffer M, Demmrich J, et al. Puncture track metastasis after ultrasound-guided fine-needle puncture biopsy. A rare complication? Dtsch Med Wochenschr 1994; 115:212–215.
61. Mazzaglia PF. Radiographic evaluation of nonfunctioning adrenal neoplasms. Surg Clin N Am 2014; 94:625–642.
62. Grumbach MM, Biller BM, Braunstein GD, et al. Management of the clinically inapparent adrenal mass ('incidentaloma'). Ann Intern Med 2003; 138:424–9.
63. Choyke PL, ACR Committee on Appropriateness Criteria. ACR Appropriateness Criteria on incidentally discovered adrenal mass. J Am Coll Radiol 2006; 3:498–504.
64. Berland LL, Silverman SG, Gore RM, et al. Managing incidental findings on abdominal CT: white paper of the ACR incidental findings committee. J Am Coll Radiol 2010; 7:754–73.
65. Walz M, Petersenn S, Koch J, et al. Endoscopic treatment of large primary adrenal tumours. Br J Surg 2005; 92:719–23.
66. Satoh F, Morimoto R, Seiji K, et al. Is there a role for segmental adrenal venous sampling and adrenal sparing surgery in patients with primary aldosteronism? Eur J Endocrinol 2015; 173:465–477.
67. Muth A, Ragnarsson O, Johannsson G, et al. Systematic review of surgery and outcomes in patients with primary aldosteronism. Br J Surg 2015; 102:307–17.
68. Citton M, Viel G, Rossi GP, et al. Outcome of surgical treatment of primary aldosteronism. Langenbecks Arch Surg 2015; 400:325–331.
69. Sancho J, Triponez F, Montet X, et al. Surgical management of adrenal metastases. Langenbecks Arch Surg 2012; 397:179–94

70. Strong VE, Kennedy T, Al-Ahmadie H, et al. Prognostic indicators of malignancy in adrenal pheochromocytomas: clinical, histopathologic, and cell cycle/apoptosis gene expression analysis. Surgery 2008; 143:759–768.
71. Thompson LD. Pheochromocytoma of the Adrenal gland Scaled Score (PASS) to separate benign from malignant neoplasms: a clinicopathologic and immunophenotypic study of 100 cases. Am J Surg Pathol 2002; 26:551–566.
72. Wu D, Tischler AS, Lloyd RV, et al. Observer variation in the application of the Pheochromocytoma of the Adrenal gland Scaled Score. Am J Surg Pathol 2009; 33:599–608.
73. Moonim MT, Johnson SJ, McNicol AM. Cancer dataset for the histological reporting of adrenal cortical carcinoma and phaeochromocytoma/paraganglioma (2nd ed). London: Royal College of Pathologists, 2012.
74. Weiss LM, Medeiros LJ, Vickery A Jr. Pathologic features of prognostic significance in adrenocortical carcinoma. Am J Surg Pathol 1989; 13:202–206.
75. Hermsen IG, Fassnacht M, Terzolo M. Plasma concentrations of o,p'DDD, o,p'DDA, and o,p'DDE as predictors of tumor response to mitotane in adrenocortical carcinoma: results of a retrospective ENS@T multicenter study. J Clin Endocrinol Metab 2011; 96:1844–51.
76. Gagner M, Lacroix A, Bolté E. Laparoscopic adrenalectomy in Cushing's syndrome and pheochromocytoma. N Engl J Med 1992; 327:1033.
77. Gaur DD. Laparoscopic operative retroperitoneoscopy: use of a new device. J Urol 1992; 148:1137–1139.
78. Walz M, Peitgen K, Hoermann R, et al. Posterior retroperitoneoscopy as a new minimally invasive approach for adrenalectomy: results of 30 adrenalectomies in 27 patients. World J Surg 1996; 20:769–74.
79. Barczyński M, Konturek A, Gołkowski F, et al. Posterior retroperitoneoscopic adrenalectomy: a comparison between the initial experience in the invention phase and introductory phase of the new surgical technique. World J Surg 2007; 31:65–71.
80. Constantinides VA, Christakis I, Touska P, et al. Systematic review and meta-analysis of retroperitoneoscopic versus laparoscopic adrenalectomy. Br J Surg 2012; 99:1639–1648.
81. Palazzo FF, Dickinson A, Phillips B, et al. Adrenal surgery in England: better outcomes in high volume practices. Clin Endocrinol (Oxf) 2016; 85:17–20.

Chapter 6

Advances in the management of neuroendocrine tumours

Jeannie F Todd, Sarah N Ali

INTRODUCTION

Neuroendocrine cells containing neurotransmitters, neuromodulators or neuropeptide hormones form a diffuse neuroendocrine system throughout the body [1]. Neuroendocrine tumours (NETs) originate from these neuroendocrine cells and are principally found within the gut (75%), but also the pancreatic islet cells (5%), lung (15%) and other organs, such as the thyroid [1].

The incidence of NETs is approximately 3 per 100,000 per year [1]. Over the last 20 years, there has been a steady increase in incidence of NETs, together with an increase in physician awareness and improvements in diagnostic techniques. Despite this, the management of patients with advanced NETs has remained challenging, due mainly to delayed diagnosis and limited therapeutic treatment options. Delayed diagnosis is often a reflection of the fact that the majority of NETs are not associated with specific symptomatology or a distinct hormonal syndrome, rather than simply a failure to detect these tumours.

At present, NETs are only curable by surgical excision of the primary tumour and/or local lymph nodes. Surgery is in most cases still the first line treatment, however the decision to operate is dependent on the stage of disease. As most of these patients present late with metastatic disease, curative surgery is often not feasible and in order to slow disease progression and for symptomatic control, patients often require medical therapies. In some cases, this may constitute systemic chemotherapy to limit tumour progression.

In order to improve outcomes, research is focussing on enhancing diagnostic tools and developing further treatment strategies, which include the already widely used somatostatin analogues, as well as biological agents.

This chapter discusses the improvements that have recently been made in diagnostic techniques and treatment for tumour and symptom control in patients with NETs.

Jeannie Todd BSc MBBS MD FRCP, Imperial Centre for Endocrinology, Imperial College Healthcare NHS Trust, Hammersmith Hospital, London, UK. Email: jeannie.todd@imperial.ac.uk (for correspondence).

Sarah N Ali BSc BM BCh (Oxon) MRCP, Imperial Centre for Endocrinology, Imperial College Healthcare NHS Trust, Hammersmith Hospital, London, UK.

CLASSIFICATION

Before discussing these advances, it is important to highlight the classification of NETs. Since 1963, NETs have been described in various classifications, primarily by their origin (foregut, midgut and hindgut) [2]. However, these classifications do not reflect biologically relevant differences in tumours, hence the trend is now to classify these tumours according to the location of the primary site (e.g. pancreas, duodenum, lung and so forth) as well as according to their functionality (e.g. gastrinoma, insulinoma) [3]. In addition, it is important to recognise that NETs may be functioning or nonfunctioning according to whether a secreted hormone is detectable and whether the distinct hormonal syndromes or associated symptoms are present [1].

The majority of NETs do not secrete excess hormones and are therefore not associated with a distinct hormonal syndrome. As such, these tumours are referred to as non-functioning NETs. These individuals often present late with nonspecific symptoms, advanced disease and poorer prognoses [4]. Conversely, functioning NETs produce excessive autonomous hormone secretion and these patients develop distinct clinical syndromes [5]. Examples include hypoglycaemia and weight gain produced by insulin release from insulinomas and flushing, diarrhoea and wheezing in carcinoid syndrome produced by release of serotonin and tachykinins from carcinoid tumours.

Aetiology

The aetiology of NETs is poorly understood. Most NETs are sporadic, but epidemiological studies show a small increased familial risk for small intestinal and colon NETs [1]. These tumours most likely result from a series of genetic mutations leading to the activation of oncogenes and/or inactivation of tumour suppressor genes and failure of apoptosis. Certainly a number of genes have been identified with the formation of NETs, such as *MEN1*, *RET*, *VHL*, *TSC1* and *TSC2*.

It is important to mention that NETs overexpress somatostatin receptors (SSTR) on the extracellular surface of the tumour [3]. This unique feature has provided a target for imaging and treatment with radiolabelled somatostatin analogues agent.

Somatostatin is an endogenous cyclic tetradecapeptide hormone, which inhibits the release of several other hormones, including serotonin, insulin, glucagon and gastrin. In addition to acting as a neurotransmitter in the gastrointestinal (GI) tract, somatostatin inhibits exocrine secretion, gastric emptying and gallbladder contraction as well as inhibiting the secretion of insulin and glucagon from the pancreas. Somatostatin binds to five subtypes of G-protein coupled transmembrane receptors (somatostatin receptors) [1-5], which are widely distributed throughout the central nervous system and the periphery. In particular, the predominant subtypes in endocrine tissues are SSTR2 and SSTR5 [6].

Diagnosis of NETs is made by the presence of clinical symptoms and syndromes, biochemical markers, radiological and nuclear imaging and/or histology [3]. Many of the clinical symptoms and biochemical markers are well understood and established, whereas developments have been made in imaging modalities and management strategies, which will be covered in this chapter.

Imaging

Whilst CT and MRI are invaluable for defining disease localisation and staging, they do not give information about tumour functionality. In addition, sensitivity of these imaging modalities to detect NETs varies from 50 to 80% depending on anatomical characteristics [7]. Functional imaging modalities, such as positron emission tomography (PET), single-photon emission computed tomography (SPECT) or scintigraphy have higher sensitivity and specificity in visualising primary tumours and their metastases [8].

Combining imaging modalities, such as PET, SPECT and scintigraphy with radiolabelled somatostatin analogues, has led to advances in nuclear medicine imaging. This field is also known as molecular imaging and achieves improvements in both diagnostic and treatment paradigms in patients with neuroendocrine tumours.

One such example of molecular imaging is the somatostatin receptor scintigraphy (SRS) [^{111}In-DTPA^0]-octreotide, also known as the OctreoScan. The OctreoScan consists of octreotide, a somatostatin analogue, the chelator DTPA and the radionuclide indium-111.

Octreotide is a synthetically modified somatostatin analogue with a longer half-life. Radioactive somatostatin analogues, such as [^{111}In-DTPA^0]-octreotide bind with high affinity to the two most prevalent somatostatin receptors, SSTR2 and SSTR5 [3]. Several studies have reported sensitivity between 67 to 100% in NET imaging with OctreoScan [9-11]. OctreoScan can be used additionally not only in the diagnosis of NETs but also in the follow-up of patients, to measure the response to treatment as well as predict the efficacy of peptide receptor radionuclide therapy (PRRT) for patients with inoperable and/or metastatic disease [12]. The OctreoScan is part of the diagnostic pathway in the European Neuroendocrine Tumour Society consensus guidelines [13,14].

There are still tumours such as primary sympathetic paragangliomas which may not be picked up by the OctreoScan, and others may not be detected because of tumour de-differentiation and some NETs. In addition, γ-imaging using ^{111}In-octreotide is limited by decreased image quality, increased physiological uptake which restricts detection of small lesions and relatively high radiation dose to the patients [15].

Therefore efforts are being made to developing further radiolabelled somatostatin analogues in order to provide higher imaging sensitivity and specificity.

Imaging with fluorine-18 fluorodeoxyglucose (FDG) PET, performed by injecting radioactive glucose, is a valuable imaging option in some cases [16]. These scans work on the principle that tumours that grow more rapidly utilise more glucose and hence FDG-avid tumours represent tumours with malignant potential as opposed to the nonavid benign tumours.

A further radioisotope uptake method involves using ^{123}I-metaiodobenzylguanidine (^{123}I-MIBG), which is taken up into active NET cells by noradrenaline transporters and stored in neurosecretory granules [3]. This method is particularly useful in patients with suspected phaeochromocytomas and paraganglioma (**Figures 6.1 to 6.3**). However, the spatial resolution of MIBG imaging is low and has limitations similar to OctreoScan [15].

Somatostatin receptor imaging can now also be performed together with PET [15]. This offers higher resolution, three-dimensional and more rapid imaging. This has been achieved by combining a generator-produced radionuclide gallium-68, with the chelator DOTA to form a stable complex with a somatostatin analogue [3]. Examples of this include [^{68}Ga]-DOTATOC and [^{68}Ga]-DOTATATE.

These ^{68}Ga-based PET scans have excellent image quality with better spatial resolution compared with imaging with γ-emitting analogues (**Figures 6.4 and 6.5**). Several of the ^{68}Ga-labelled somatostatin analogues have been evaluated for PET scanning of NETs and have shown higher sensitivity and specificity compared with the [^{111}In-DTPA^0]-octreotide scintigraphy [17,18].

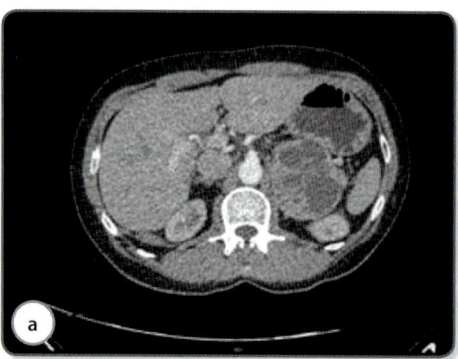 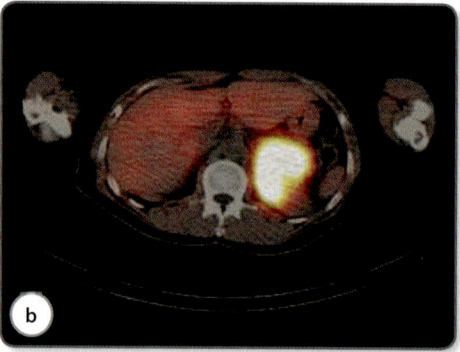

Figure 6.1 (a) CT imaging and (b) [^{123}I]-MIBG imaging with SPECT of a left adrenal phaeochromocytoma.

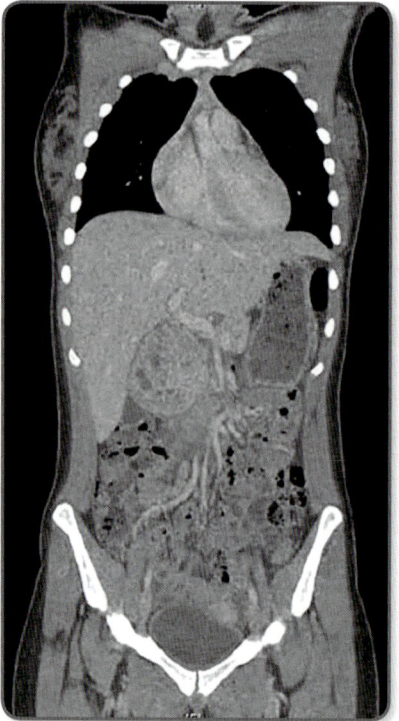 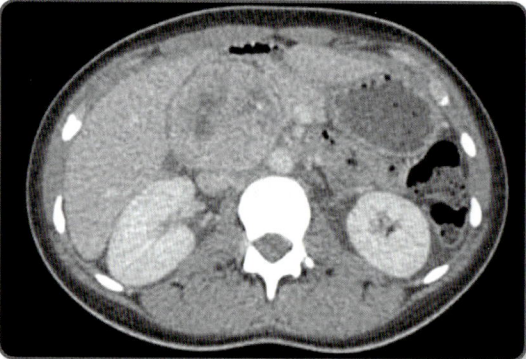

Figure 6.2 CT imaging of a large anterior paraganglioma.

These [^{68}Ga]-based PET scans are currently only available at specialist centres and may replace SRS due to higher sensitivity and ease of administration [3].

[^{68}Ga]-DOTATATE PET/CT has demonstrated superiority in spatial resolution and lesion detection compared to OctreoScan, MIBG scintigraphy and MRI [19,20]. In addition, [^{68}Ga]-DOTATATE is more convenient to patients as it can be completed in less than 2 hours versus 2 days for OctreoScan or MIBG imaging, as well as involving lower radiation exposure [15].

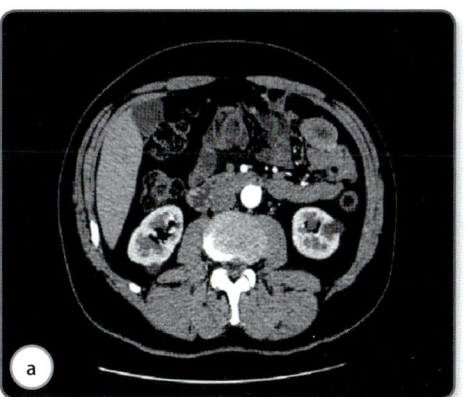

Figure 6.3 [^{123}I]-MIBG imaging with SPECT of a large anterior paraganglioma.

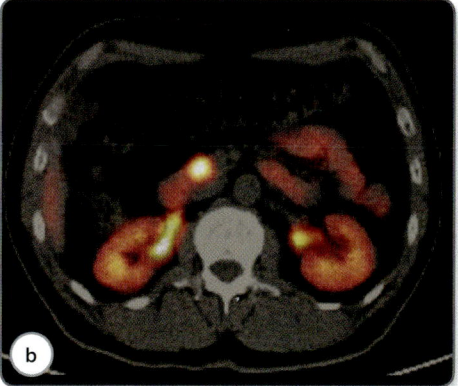

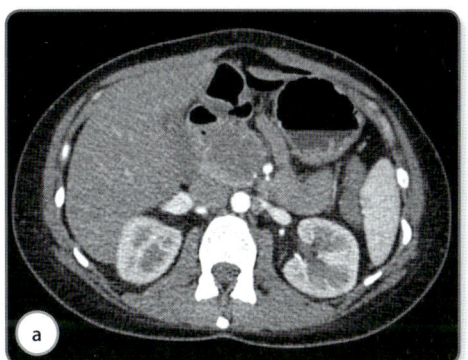

a

b

Figure 6.4 (a) CT imaging and (b) [^{68}Ga]-DOTATATE PET CT scan of an insulinoma in the head of pancreas.

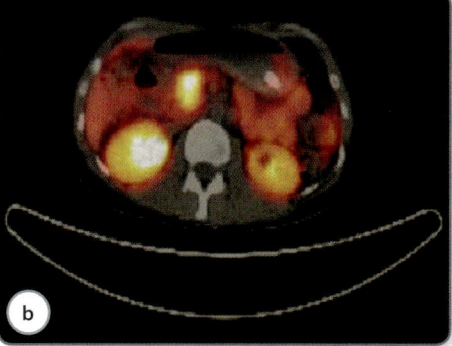

a

b

Figure 6.5 (a) CT imaging and (b) [^{68}Ga]-DOTATATE PET CT scan of a low-grade neuroendocrine tumour in the small bowel.

A meta-analysis of 14 papers, totalling 570 patients with NETs compared the sensitivity and specificity of the various imaging modalities in the diagnosis of primary or metastatic NET lesions [15]. As with previous studies, this meta-analysis showed that [68Ga]-DOTATATE PET/CT was superior to other modalities. One study analysed showed that the sensitivity of the [68Ga]-DOTATATE PET/CT in the diagnosis of primary or metastatic lesions in NETs ranged from 80–100%, with a specificity of 82–90%, compared with a specificity of the OctreoScan of 98%. In comparison, one study showed a much lower sensitivity of MIBG scintigraphy ranging from 41.6–60%, despite having a good specificity of 100% in 2 studies. Another study reported the sensitivity and specificity of the [68Ga]-DOTATATE PET/CT to be 93.8–100%, compared to 92.6 100% for MRI. Furthermore, three studies comparing [68Ga]-DOTATATE PET/CT to 18F-FDG PET/CT reported sensitivity of 72.2–100% and 66–77.8%, respectively [15].

Glucagon-like peptide 1 receptor imaging

Glucagon-like peptide 1 (GLP-1) is involved in the normal glucose homeostasis, by binding to specific receptors on the surface of pancreatic islet beta cells to stimulate glucose-induced insulin secretion. Overexpression of the GLP-1 receptor has been found on many types of cancer cells, such as benign insulinomas, gastrinomas, phaeochromocytomas and medullary thyroid cancer [21]. This finding has led to the development of scintigraphy and PET with the use of GLP-1 analogues (such as exendin-4) labelled with radioisotopes, 111In, 99mTc, 68Ga, 18F and 64Cu. Whilst there have been a number of clinical studies investigating the use of GLP-1 receptor imaging, it is not yet widely clinically available and further studies with larger numbers of patients are required to evaluate its clinical value for NETs [21-26].

ADVANCES IN MANAGEMENT OF NETS

Somatostatin analogues

Secretory NET cells express cell surface somatostatin receptors (SSTR1-5). Somatostatin and its analogues exert antitumour activity directly through binding to the somatostatin receptors on the tumour cells [27]. Activation of these receptors brings about tumour growth repression and potentially, tumour regression, by inhibition of growth factor signalling, inhibition of the cell cycle, as well as a pro-apoptotic effect on the neuroendocrine tumour [27].

This is the rationale for the development of somatostatin analogues for tumour therapy.

Octreotide was the first available somatostatin analogue. Octreotide was shown to reduce the symptoms of carcinoid syndrome and this was associated with reduced urinary 5HIAA levels [28]. A drawback to its use is its short half-life of 2 hours. The longer acting LAR formulation addresses this issue and can be administered monthly, making it the mainstay treatment for carcinoid syndrome [3].

Lanreotide is another long-acting somatostatin analogue available with a similar binding profile to octreotide and can also be administered monthly. Both Octreotide and lanreotide can control clinical symptoms in functioning NETs that predominately express SSTR2 and SSTR5 [3].

The PROMID trial is a placebo-controlled double blind phase IIIB study performed in patients with well-differentiated metastatic mid-gut neuroendocrine tumours (NETs).

This trial investigated the effects of octreotide LAR in 85 treatment-naïve patients. Patients were assigned to either placebo or octreotide LAR 30 mg administered intramuscularly monthly until tumour progression or death. The trial showed that octreotide LAR significantly lengthened the time to tumour progression compared with placebo in patients with either functionally active or inactive metastatic midgut NETs [29].

CLARINET, a large prospective Phase III trial evaluated the effects of lanreotide on 204 patients with nonfunctioning gastroenteropancreatic neuroendocrine tumours (GEP-NETs). Tumours included pancreatic and GI tumours, which were well- or moderately differentiated and stable. In 62% of patients treated with lanreotide, there was no death or disease progression compared to 22% of placebo patients over a period of 2 years [30]. An open label study on the long-term use of lanreotide is currently underway.

Some studies and clinical experience have shown however, that after about 6–18 months of octreotide/lanreotide therapy, some NETs patients may experience a loss of response. It is thought that this is principally due to an internalisation or down-regulation of the SSTR2 expression, or due to up-regulation of the other somatostatin receptors [31,32].

This limited duration of use with octreotide/lanreotide has led to the development of pasireotide (SOM230). Pasireotide is a novel multireceptor-targeted analogue with a high affinity for four out of the five somatostatin receptor subtypes. In addition, pasireotide has a 40-fold higher affinity for SSTR5 than octreotide. This coupled with the broad affinity for SSTR subtypes may therefore allow it to be of use in a wider spectrum of patients, who have not responded to octreotide and lanreotide, providing continued symptomatic relief after initial treatment failure [3,33].

A multi-centre phase II trial suggests pasireotide effectively controls diarrhoea and flushing in 27% of patients who were resistant or refractory to octreotide LAR [34]. A phase III study comparing pasireotide LAR and octreotide LAR is currently ongoing in patients with metastatic GI NETs, in whom disease related symptoms are inadequately controlled by somatostatin analogues (trial NCT00690430).

SYSTEMIC THERAPY: CHEMOTHERAPY

Many patients with metastatic NET lesions require chemotherapy to control hormonal symptoms and limit tumour progression. Single agents, such as fluorouracil, dacarbazine, doxorubicin and streptozotocin have been evaluated in patients with metastatic NETs. However, little benefit in tumour shrinkage and symptomatic relief has been shown [35]. Combination chemotherapy regimens have also been evaluated, however no regimen has yet shown a response rate greater than 15% in small intestinal NETs using the criterion of a 50% decrease in bidimensionally measurable disease [36]. A phase II/III trial with 249 patients with advanced carcinoid tumours were randomised to doxorubicin plus fluorouracil or streptozotocin plus fluorouracil. Patients received dacarbazine treatment in the event of disease progression. In the group treated with streptozotocin plus fluorouracil, a significantly longer median survival was seen (24.3 compared with 15.6 months), however there was no difference in tumour response rate between groups [37]. In patients with pancreatic NETs (pNETs), streptozotocin in combination with other agents, such as 5-fluorouracil, cisplatin, or doxorubicin, has yielded promising response rates of approximately 40% [38].

Researchers are also looking into the potential of combining these systemic chemotherapy agents with somatostatin analogues to assess whether this will allow for more specific targeting of metastatic NETs. One study has investigated the use of lanreotide together with paclitaxel and carboplastin in small-cell lung cancer patients. Those patients treated with the combination of chemotherapy and lanreotide 30 mg did have an overall better survival benefit, however, interestingly this was only significant in those patients with limited disease [39].

SYSTEMIC THERAPY: EVEROLIMUS PLUS OCTREOTIDE

Recent work has focussed on developing targeted biological therapies. One such target in NETs is the mammalian target of rapamycin (mTOR) pathway. mTOR is a central regulator of protein synthesis important in cancer development, including cell growth and proliferation, angiogenesis and cell metabolism. Although dysregulation of mTOR may not be essential in the pathogenesis of NETs, key growth factors, such as insulin-like growth factor 1 receptor and epidermal growth factor receptor, involved in tumour proliferation of NETs mediate their effects via mTOR. Hence, mTOR is a promising target.

Everolimus is a once-daily oral mTOR inhibitor, which blocks the mTOR pathway by binding to its intracellular receptor FKBP-12.

In individual cases, everolimus has been effective in high-grade tumours [3]. The RADIANT-3 trial, a phase III placebo-controlled multicentre trial compared everolimus 10 mg/day plus best supportive care (BSC) to placebo plus BSC in 410 patients with low- or intermediate-grade pNETs. The median progression-free survival was 11 months in the everolimus group compared to 4.6 months in the placebo group, resulting in a 65% reduction in the estimated risk of progression ($p < 0.001$). Although drug-related adverse effects were present, such as stomatitis, rash and diarrhoea, these were mostly mild to moderate [40].

Preclinical studies have also suggested that everolimus together with somatostatin analogues may have synergistic antitumour effects [41].

In a phase II trial, RADIANT-1, everolimus 10 mg/day was used with or without octreotide LAR < 30 mg/month in patients with advanced pNETs after chemotherapy failure. Results showed a median progression-free survival of 9.7 months in patients who received everolimus only compared to 16.7 months in those who received both everolimus and octreotide [42]. In addition, 59.3% and 84.2% of patients, receiving everolimus only and everolimus plus octreotide, respectively experienced disease stabilisation or tumour shrinkage.

RADIANT-2, a phase III, double-blind, randomised controlled trial compared everolimus plus octreotide with octreotide LAR only in patients with advanced NETs. The study showed a 23% reduction in the estimated risk of progression in patients treated with everolimus plus octreotide compared with patients who received octreotide LAR only. In addition, progression-free survival was a median of 11.3 months in the octreotide LAR only group compared with 16.4 months in the everolimus plus octreotide combination group [43].

PEPTIDE RECEPTOR RADIONUCLIDE THERAPY

Patients in whom NETs continue to grow after treatment with somatostatin analogues and may respond to systemic PRRT. This is particularly true if there has been evidence of uptake of [123I]-MIBG or [111In]-octreotide at all known tumour sites during diagnostic imaging.

By labelling somatostatin analogues with therapeutic radionuclides, such as ^{111}In, ^{90}Y, ^{177}Lu and [213]Bi, the analogues can specifically bind to SSTRs on tumour cells. In this way, these PRRTs can deliver an effective radiation dose to tumours with minimal damage to healthy tissues. This PRRT technique has been shown in a number of studies to potentially benefit patients with unresectable somatostatin receptor-positive NETs [5,44,45].

Indium-111 not only emits γ-radiation, which easily penetrates tissues and can be imaged with a γ-scanner, but also emits therapeutic Auger and conversion electrons that play an antiproliferative role in malignant tumours with a short to medium tissue penetration [46]. Although initial studies with high radioactivity doses of [^{111}In-DTPA[0]]-octreotide in patients with metastatic NETs resulted in significant symptom control, there were relatively few tumour responses, as a result of it not being an ideal option for PRRT due to its small particle range of Auger electrons [47–49].

In comparison, yttrium-90 is a beta-particle emitter, which combined with a more stable chelator DOTA and a modified SST analogue octreotide, gives a tracer [^{90}Y]-DOTATOC. This has a superior therapeutic efficacy compared to [^{111}In-DTPA[0]]-octreotide to cause cell damage and is generally well tolerated [50].

In three small studies, treatment with [^{90}Y]-DOTATOC was associated with 7–31% complete or partial response rates and 23–74% stable disease rates in patients with NETs [51] [^{90}Y]-DOTATOC has been shown to improve symptoms, including diarrhoea in 90 patients with metastatic NETs of the GI tract and bronchus, with improved progression-free survival of 18.2 versus 7.9 months; $p = 0.03$ [52].

Another study investigating 116 patients with metastatic NETs undergoing PRRT with [^{90}Y]-DOTATOC found a response rate in 31 patients (26%) including complete remission in 4% and partial remission in 22%. 72 patients (62%) showed stabilisation of their diseases, however in the remaining patients (11%) the disease continued to progress. Encouragingly, the radionuclide was well tolerated, with no serious side effects reported [53].

Similarly, a phase II study of 41 patients with GEP-NETs and bronchial tumours were given four intravenous injections of ^{90}Y radionuclide therapy. The results of this study showed a tumour response rate of 24%, with complete response in 2% of patients and partial remission in 22% of patients. 5% of patients suffered from grade III pancytopenia, which was the most severe adverse event [54].

In a larger study, 1109 patients from 29 countries were treated with repeated cycles of [^{90}Y]-DOTATOC. Tumour response was seen in 34.1% (378 patients), with 5.2% (58 patients) achieving stable disease. The median survival from diagnosis was 94.6 months, which was longer than the expected median survival of 33 months survival. Longer survival was associated with morphological, biochemical and clinical response, as well as high tumour uptake in pre-therapeutic somatostatin receptor scintigraphy [55]. However, severe haematological and permanent renal toxicity occurred in 143 (12.9%) and 102 (9.2%) patients, respectively. Despite differences in protocols, it appears that the therapeutic effect of [^{90}Y]-DOTATOC is seen in approximately 20–28% of patients with NETs and 28–38% in patients with GEP-NETs [56].

More recent advances in radionuclide therapy involve the radiolabelled somatostatin analogue [^{177}Lu]-DOTA[0] Tyr[3]-octreotate ([^{177}Lu]-DOTATATE). Lutetium-177 is a median energy B-emitter with a small particle range allowing for a higher radiation dose to be delivered to smaller tumours and with less damage to surrounding tissues than the radionuclide [90]Y [57]. Lutetium-177 also emits γ-rays, thus these radionuclides can be used for treatment as well as for dosimetry and monitoring of tumour response.

Radionuclide therapy with lutetium-177 was introduced more than a decade ago for targeted treatment of advanced GEP-NETs in the form of [^{177}Lu]-octreotate, which attaches onto the overexpressed and upregulated somatostatin receptors on these well-differentiated tumours [58]. PRRT with [^{177}Lu]-octreotate has since been shown to be effective and safe in many small clinical trials, although the absence of randomised controlled trials of [^{177}Lu]-octreotate has precluded acceptance of PRRT in mainstream oncology practice [59].

Looking at these earlier small trials, one study which compared [^{177}Lu]-DOTATATE with [^{111}In-DTPA^0]-octreotide in 6 patients with SSTR positive tumours showed that after 24 hours, the uptake of [^{177}Lu]-DOTATATE was almost equal to [^{111}In-DTPA^0]-octreotide for the kidneys, however 3- to 4-fold higher in four of the analysed tumours. This suggests that [^{177}Lu]-DOTATATE represents a targeted tumour treatment [60].

Another trial assessing PRRT with the [^{177}Lu]-DOTATATE in 310 NET patients showed complete and partial tumour remission in 2% and 28%, respectively. In addition, 16% of patients treated with [^{177}Lu]-DOTATATE had a minor tumour response (decrease of >25% to <50% in size) [58].

Further larger randomised controlled trials of [^{177}Lu]-octreotate PRRT are underway, but phase II studies over the past decade have demonstrated a clinically beneficial response in 25% of GEP-NET patients [58] with stabilisation of progressive disease and progression-free survival of approximately 3 years [58,61,62].

In addition, a phase I study (NETTLE) has combined treatment with [^{177}Lu]-octreotate and the systemic biological agent, everolimus as a PRRT in advanced progressive GEP-NETs [63]. This study has shown that the overall tumour response rate was 44% (7 of 16 patients), and no patient's neuroendocrine lesion progressed over the 6-month period of treatment. 4 of 5 pancreatic NET patients achieved a partial response of 80% and no patient suffered from tumour progression during the study. Toxicity was observed at all dosage levels of everolimus, but they appear manageable and reversible. All patients required dose reduction or complete cessation of everolimus at the 10-mg level, because of therapy induced neutropenia and thrombocytopenia, and reduced creatinine clearance. Renal impairment occurred with everolimus doses above 7.5 mg and was dose limiting. This shows promise that everolimus may be combined safely with [^{177}Lu]-octreotate to treat low-grade NETs [63]. A phase II study is awaited.

CONCLUSION

The incidence of NETs has been steadily increasing with many patients presenting late, often with metastatic disease. As a result, surgical intervention, although valuable is often not curative. The use of somatostatin analogues has become a mainstay in the management of symptoms in many patients with NETs. Newer combinations of everolimus and somatostatin analogues and radionuclide therapies may provide promising future treatments for the prolongation of time to disease progression and improved survival outcomes.

Key points for clinical practice

- The incidence of NETs is increasing. Most patients present late, often with metastatic disease.
- Whilst surgical resection is often still first line, medical treatments, including systemic chemotherapy, are helpful with symptom control and disease progression.
- Secretory NET cells overexpress somatostatin receptors and therefore, somatostatin analogues have become a mainstay in the management of symptomatic control.
- Newer combinations of systemic chemotherapy (everolimus) and somatostatin analogues, and radionuclide therapies provide promising future treatments for the prolongation of time to disease progression and improved survival outcomes.
- Molecular imaging, which combines imaging modalities, such as PET, SPECT and scintigraphy with radiolabelled somatostatin analogues, has achieved improvements in both diagnostic and treatment paradigms in patients with neuroendocrine tumours.

REFERENCES

1. Sam A, Meeran K. Chapter 32: Neuroendocrine tumours. Lecture Notes: Endocrinology and Diabetes. Chichester: Wiley-Blackwell, 2009.
2. Williams ED, Sandler M. The classification of carcinoid tumours. Lancet 1963; 1:238–239.
3. Oberg KE. The Management of Neuroendocrine Tumours: Current and Future Medical Therapy Options. Clin Oncol (R Coll Radiol) 2010; 24:282–293.
4. Metz DC, Jensen RT. Gastrointestinal neuroendocrine tumours: pancreatic endocrine tumours. Gastroenterology 2008; 135:1469–1492.
5. Ramage JK, Davies AH, Ardil J, et al. Guidelines for the management of gastroenteropancreatic neuroendocrine (including carcinoid) tumours. Gut 2005; 449:395–401.
6. Barnett P. Somatostatin and somatostatin receptor physiology. Endocrine 2003; 20:255–264.
7. Wong KK, Waterfield RT, Marzola MC, et al. Contemporary nuclear medicine imaging of neuroendocrine tumours. Clin Radiol 2012; 67:1035–1050.
8. Xu C, Zhang H. Somatostatin receptor-based imaging and radionuclide therapy. BioMed Res Int 2015; 2015:1–14.
9. Srirajakanthan R, Kayani I, Quigley AM, et al. The role of ^{68}Ga-DOTATATE PET in patients with neuroendocrine tumours and negative or equivocal findings on ^{111}In-DTPA-octreotide scintigraphy. J Nucl Med 2010; 51:875–882.
10. Hildebrandt G, Scheidhauer K, Luyken C, et al. High sensitivity of the in vivo detection of somatostatin receptors by [111]Indium (DTPA-octreotide)-scintigraphy in meningioma patients. Acta Neurochir (Wien) 1994; 126:63–71.
11. Lebtahi R, Le Cloirec J, Houzard C, et al. Detection of neuro-endocrine tumours. 99mTc-P829 scintigraphy compared with ^{111}In-pentetreotide scintigraphy. J Nucl Med 2002; 43:889–895.
12. Bombardieri E, Ambrosini V, Aktolun C, et al. ^{111}In-pentetreotide scintigraphy procedure guidelines for tumour imaging. Eur J Nucl Med Mol Imaging 2010; 37:1441–1448.
13. Pavel M, Baudin E, Couvelard A, et al. ENETS consensus guidelines for the management of patients with liver and other distant metastases from neuroendocrine neoplasms of foregut, midgut, hindgut and unknown primary. Neuroendocrinology 2012; 95:157–176.
14. Pape UF, Perren A, Niederle B, et al. ENETS consensus guidelines for the management of patients with neuroendocrine neoplasms from the jejuno-ileum and the appendix including goblet cell carcinomas. Neuroendocrinology 2012; 95:135–156.
15. Mojtahedi A, Thamake S, Tworowska I, et al. The value of ^{68}Ga-DOTATATE PET/CT in diagnosis and management of neuroendocrine tumors compared to current FDA approved imaging modalities: a review of literature. Am J Nucl Med Mol Imaging 2014; 4:426–434.

16. Hofman MS, Hicks RJ. Changing paradigms with molecular imaging of neuroendocrine tumours. Discov Med 2012; 14:71–81.

17. Hofman MS, Kong G, Neels OC, et al. High management impact of Ga-68 DOTATATE (GaTate) PET/CT for imaging neuroendocrine and other somatostatin expressing tumours. J Med Imaging Radiat Oncol 2012; 56:40–47.

18. Kayani I, Bomanji JB, Groves A, et al. Functional imaging of neuroendocrine tumours with combined PET/CT using (68)Gallium DOTATATE (DOTA-DPhe1, Tyr3-octreotate) and 18F-FDG. Cancer 2008; 112:2447–2455.

19. Antunes P, Ginj M, Zhang H, et al. Are radio gallium labelled DOTA-conjugated somatostatin analogues superior to those labelled with other radiometals? Eur J Nucl Med Mol Imaging 2007; 34:982–993.

20. Poeppel TD, Binse I, Petersenn S, et al. 68Ga-DOTATOC versus 68Ga-DOTATATE PET/CT in functional imaging of neuroendocrine tumors. J Nucl Med 2011; 52:1864–1870.

21. Hubalewska-Dydejczyk A, Sowa-Staszczak A, Tomaszuk M, et al. GLP-1 and exendin-4 for imaging endocrine pancreas. A review. Labelled glucagon-like peptide-1 analogues: past, present and future. Q J Nucl Med Mol Imaging. 2015; 59:152–160.

22. Gotthardt M, Lalyko G, van Eerd-Vismale J, et al. A new technique for in vivo imaging of specific GLP-1 binding sites: first results in small rodents. Regul Pept 2006; 137:162–167.

23. Wild D, Mäcke H, Christ E, et al. Glucagon-like peptide 1-receptor scans to localize occult insulinomas. N Engl J Med 2008; 359:766–768.

24. Sowa-Staszczak A, Pach D, Mikołajczak R, et al. Glucagon-like peptide-1 receptor imaging with [Lys40(Ahx-HYNIC-99mTc/EDDA)NH2]-exendin-4 for the detection of insulinoma. Eur J Nucl Med Mol Imaging 2013; 40:524–531.

25. Reubi JC, Waser B. Concomitant expression of several peptide receptors in neuroendocrine tumours: molecular basis for in vivo multireceptor tumour targeting. Eur J Nucl Med Mol Imaging 2003; 30:781–793.

26. Selvaraju RK, Velikyan I, Johansson L, et al. In vivo imaging of the glucagonlike peptide 1 receptor in the pancreas with 68Ga-labeled DO3A-exendin-4. J Nucl Med 2013; 54:1458–1463.

27. Rai U, Thrimawithana TR, Valery C, et al. Therapeutic uses of somatostatin and its analogues: Current view and potential applications. Pharmacology & Therapeutics 2015; 152:98–110.

28. Susini C, Buscail L. Rationale for the use of somatostatin analogs as antitumour agents. Ann Oncol 2006; 17:1733–1742.

29. Rinke A, Muller HH, Schade-Brittinger C, et al. Placebo-controlled, double blind, prospective, randomised study on the effect of octreotide LAR in the control of tumour growth in patients with metastatic neuroendocrine midgut tumours: a report from the PROMID study group. J Clin Oncol 2009; 27:4656–4663.

30. Caplin M, Ruszniewski P, Pavel M, et al. A randomised, double-blind, placebo-Controlled study of Lanreotide Antiproliferative Response In patients with gastroenteropancreatic NeuroEndocrine Tumours (CLARINET), the European Cancer Congress 2013.

31. Hofland LJ, van der Hoek J, Feelders R, et al. Pre-clinical and clinical experiences with novel somatostatin ligands: advantages, disadvantages and new prospects. J Endocrinol Invest 2005; 28:36–40.

32. van Vugt HH, Smid HA, Sailer AW. Ligand-dependent internalization of somatostatin receptors. Endocr Abstracts 2008; 16:P659.

33. Schmid HA. Pasireotide (SOM230): development, mechanism of action and potential applications. Mol Cell Endocrinol 2008; 286:69–74.

34. Kvols L, Oberg KE, O'Dorisio TM, et al. Pasireotide (SOM230) shows efficacy and tolerability in the treatment of patients with advanced neuroendocrine tumours refractory or resistant to octreotide LER: results of a phase II study. Endocr Relat Cancer 2012; 19:657–666.

35. Moertel CG. Treatment of the carcinoid tumour and the malignant carcinoid syndrome. J Clin Oncol 1983; 1:727–740.

36. Schnire II, Yao JC, Ajani JA. Carcinoid – a comprehensive review. Acta 2003; 42:672–692.

37. Sun W, Lipsitz S, Catalano P, et al. Phase II/III study of doxorubicin with fluorouracil compared with streptozotocin with fluorouracil or dacarbazine in the treatment of advanced carcinoid tumours. Eastern Cooperative Oncology Group Study E1281. J Clin Oncol 2005; 23:4897–4904.

38. Modlin IM, Latich I, Kidd M, et al. Therapeutic options for gastrointestinal carcinoids. Clin Gastroenterol Hepatol 2006; 4:526–547.

39. Zarogoulidis K, Eleftheriadou E, Kontakiotis T, et al. Long acting somatostatin analogues in combination to antineoplastic agents in the treatment of small cell lung cancer patients. Lung Cancer 2012; 76:84–88.

40. Yao JC, Shah MH, Ito T, et al. Everolimus for advanced pancreatic neuroendocrine tumours. N Engl J Med 2011; 364:514–523.

41. Grozinsky-Glasberg S, Shimon I, Korbonits M, et al. Somatostatin analogues in the control of neuroendocrine tumours: efficacy and mechanisms. Endocr Relat Cancer 2008; 15:701–720.
42. Yao JC, Lombard-Bohas C, Baudin E, et al. Daily oral everolimus activity in patients with metastatic pancreatic neuroendocrine tumours after failure of cytotoxic chemotherapy; a phase II trial. J Clin Oncol 2010; 28:69–76.
43. Pavel ME, Hainsworth JD, Baudin E, et al. Everolimus plus octreotide long acting repeatable for the treatment of advanced neuroendocrine tumours associated with carcinoid syndrome (RADIANT-2): a randomised, placebo-controlled, phase 3 study. Lancet 2011; 378:2005–2012.
44. Comaru-Schally AM, Schally AV. A clinical overview of carcinoid tumours: perspective for improvement in treatment using peptide analogs (review). Int J Oncol 2005; 26:301–309.
45. Forrer F, Valkema R, Kwekkeboom DJ, et al. Neuroendocrine tumours: peptide receptor radionuclide therapy. Best Pract Res Clin Endocrinol Metab 2007; 21:111–129.
46. Krenning EP, de Jong M, Kooij PP, et al. Radiolabelled somatostatin analogues for peptide receptor scintigraphy and radionuclide therapy. Ann Oncol 1999; 10; S23–S29.
47. Anthony LB, Woltering EA, Espenan GD, et al. Indium-111-pentetreotide prolongs survival in gastroenteropancreatic malignancies. Semin Nucl Med 2002; 32:123–132.
48. Delpassand ES, Sims-Mourtada J, Saso H, et al. Safety and efficacy of radionuclide therapy with high-activity In-111 pentetreotide in patients with progressive neuroendocrine tumors. Cancer Biother Radiopharm 2008; 23:292–300.
49. Capello A, Krenning EP, Breeman WA, et al. Peptide receptor radionuclide therapy in vitro using [111In-DTPA^0]-octreotide. J Nucl Med 2003; 44:98–104.
50. Bodei L, Cremonesi M, Grana CM, et al. Yttrium-labelled peptides for therapy of NET. Eur J Nucl Med Mol Imaging 2012; 39:S93–102.
51. Kaltsas GA, Papadogias D, Makras P, et al. Treatment of advanced neuroendocrine tumours with radiolabelled somatostatin analogues. Endocr Relat Cancer 2005; 12:683–699.
52. Bushnell Jr DL, O'Dorisio TM, O'Dorisio MS, et al. 90Y-Edotreotide for metastatic carcinoid refractory to octreotide. J Clin Oncol 2010; 28:1652–1659.
53. Forrer E, Waldherr C, Maecke HR, et al. Targeted radionuclide therapy with 90Y-DOTATOC in patients with neuroendocrine tumours. Anticancer Research 2006; 20:703–707.
54. Waldherr C, Pless M, Maecke HR, et al. The clinical value of [90Y-DOTA]-D-Phe1-Tyr3-octreotide (90Y-DOTATOC) in the treatment of neuroendocrine tumours: a clinical phase II study. Ann Oncol 2001; 12:941–945.
55. Imhof A, Brunner P, Marincek N, et al. Response, survival, and long-term toxicity after therapy with the radiolabeled somatostatin analogue [90Y-DOTA]-TOC in metastasized neuroendocrine cancers. J Clin Oncol 2011; 29:2416–2423.
56. Nisa L, Savelli G, Giubbini R. Yttrium-90 DOTATOC therapy in GEP-NET and other SST2 expressing tumors: a selected review. Ann Nucl Med 2011; 25:75–85.
57. Romer A, Seiler D, Marincek N, et al. Somatostatin-based radiopeptide therapy with [177Lu-DOTA]-TOC versus [90Y-DOTA]-TOC in neuroendocrine tumours. Eur J Nucl Med Mol Imaging 2014; 41:214–222.
58. Kwekkeboom DJ, de Herder WW, Kam BL, et al. Treatment with the radiolabelled somatostatin analog [177 Lu-DOTA0, Tyr3]-octreotate: toxicity, efficacy, and survival. J Clin Oncol 2008; 26:2124–2130.
59. Jensen RT, Cadiot G, Brandi ML, et al. ENETS Consensus Guidelines for the management of patients with digestive neuroendocrine neoplasms: Functional pancreatic endocrine tumor syndromes. Neuroendocrinology 2012; 95:98.
60. Kwekkeboom DJ, Bakker WH, Kooij PP, et al. [177Lu-DOTAO-Tyr3]-octreotate: comparison with [111In-DTPA^0]-octreotide in patients. Eur J Nucl Med 2001; 28:1319–1325.
61. Jan H, Wyld D, Burge M. Efficacy of PRRT in Metastatic Neuroendocrine Tumors; A retrospective large single institutional study. ENETS 12th Annual Conference Proc 2015; 102:136 (Abst N3).
62. Ezziddin S, Attassi M, Yong-Hing CJ, et al. Predictors of long-term outcome in patients with well differentiated gastroenteropancreatic neuroendocrine tumors after peptide receptor radionuclide therapy with 177Lu-octreotate. J Nucl Med 2014; 55:183.
63. Claringbold PG, Turner JH. NeuroEndocrine Tumor Therapy with Lutetium-177-octreotate and Everolimus (NETTLE): A Phase I Study. Cancer Biother Radiopharm 2015; 30:261–269.

Chapter 7

Male infertility

Riada McCredie, Thomas Brenton, Jonathan WA Ramsay, Channa N Jayasena

INTRODUCTION

Infertility is defined by the World Health Organization (WHO) [1] as a failure to conceive a clinical pregnancy after 12 months or more of regular unprotected sexual intercourse, and is based on observing that 84% of couples will conceive after 1 year, 92% after 2 years and 93% after 3 years [2]. One third of infertility is reported as being due to the male partner, but the true extent of male infertility is likely to be underestimated. In 2014, on average 25.4% of patients at UK fertility clinics were undergoing treatment for male factor infertility and 11.5% for mixed male and female factor infertility [3]. The probability of natural conception is related to the total number of motile sperm in the ejaculate. Men with a sperm concentration in the bottom 5% of the population (defined as < 15 million sperm per mL by the WHO) [4], are oligospermic. Men with less than 40% sperm motility in the ejaculate are asthenospermic. Men with low levels of androgen have hypogonadism. This chapter will discuss the major aetiological factors in male infertility and hypogonadism, and then discuss approaches to managing affected patients.

PHYSIOLOGY OF MALE FERTILITY

Male fertility is orchestrated by the hypothalamic-pituitary-gonadal axis [5] (**Figure 7.1**). The median eminence of the hypothalamus releases gonadotrophin-releasing hormone (GnRH) to the portal circulation in a pulsatile manner, which stimulates the anterior pituitary to secrete pulses of the gonadotrophin hormones, luteinising hormone (LH) and follicle stimulating hormone (FSH). LH stimulates the testicular Leydig cells to synthesise testosterone, and FSH stimulates Sertoli cells in the seminiferous tubules to support spermatogenesis. LH and FSH levels are negatively regulated by testosterone and inhibin, respectively. An entire cycle of spermatogenesis lasts on average 64 days[6].

Channa N. Jayasena PhD MRCP FRCPath, Department of Andrology, Hammersmith Hospital, London, UK. Email: c.jayasena@imperial.ac.uk (for correspondence).

Riada McCredie BMSc (Hons) MBChB (Hons), Department of Andrology, Hammersmith Hospital, London, UK.

Thomas Brenton BSc (Hons) BMBS MRCS, Department of Andrology, Hammersmith Hospital, London, UK.

Jonathan WA Ramsay MS FRC (Urol) Imperial College Healthcare Trust, London, UK.

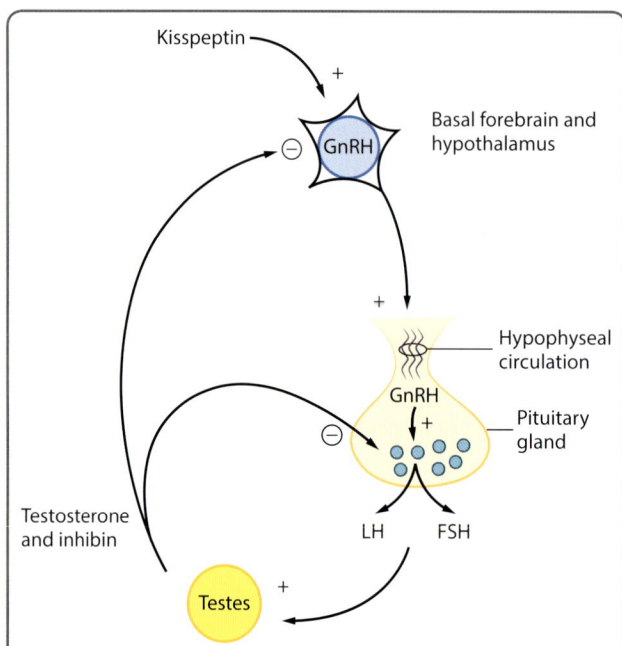

Figure 7.1 The male hypothalamo-pituitary-gonadal axis.

AETIOLOGY OF MALE INFERTILITY

For the purposes of this chapter, the causes of male infertility [7-11] have been broadly sub-divided into testicular failure, obstructive male infertility (more commonly termed obstructive azoospermia) and hypothalamo-pituitary disease. However, male factor infertility may be multifactorial and both male and female factor components to infertility may be present.

TESTICULAR FAILURE

Primary testicular failure classically results in low testosterone, high LH and FSH secretion and oligoasthenospermia or azoospermia associated with deficient sperm production. Azoospermia may arise from complete testicular failure associated with genetic factors, cryptorchidism, mumps orchitis, testicular cancer, radiotherapy and chemotherapy agents such as cyclophosphamide. Milder testicular failure associated with oligoasthenozoospermia may be caused by lifestyle factors or drugs [7,12,13] such as allopurinol, colchicine, sulfasalazine, cyclosporine, methotrexate, cimetidine, amiodarone, nitrofurantoin, erythromycin, carbamazepine, sodium valproate, phenytoin, calcium channel blockers and antiretroviral agents.

Lifestyle factors causing testicular failure

Obesity contributes to infertility in several ways, and is associated with a decreased total sperm count, concentration and motility. Adipocytes express the aromatase cytochrome p450 enzyme which converts androgens into oestrogen, and may suppress the pituitary secretion of FSH leading to a decrease in spermatogenesis [14]. Obesity is also linked with hyperinsulinaemia and decreased levels of sex hormone binding globulin (SHBG), which may further increase the proportion of oestrogen which is free and therefore biologically active. Obese men are also more likely to suffer sleep apnoea which disrupts the normal circadian pattern of testosterone secretion [15]. These patients may present with low levels of free and total testosterone and a decreased ratio of testosterone to oestrogen. Obesity is also associated with increased reactive oxygen species (ROS) and oxidative stress which can cause sperm DNA damage and an increased DNA fragmentation index [16]. An increase in scrotal fat can also cause an increase in scrotal temperature and the local accumulation of fat-soluble environmental toxins.

Chronic alcohol abuse impairs male fertility by decreasing semen volume, sperm concentration and motility and may be linked with reduced libido and erectile function [17]. Acute alcohol intoxication has also been associated with abnormal spermatogenesis and sperm function however it has not been proven that a moderate alcohol intake impairs fertility [13]. Smoking may decrease sperm concentration by, on average, 22% when compared with non-smokers [18]. Reduced motility and abnormal morphology have also been reported and it is proposed that these abnormal parameters are caused by ROS present in cigarette smoke.

Recreational opioid use inhibits endogenous GnRH secretion, and the sex steroid properties of cannabis may disrupt spermatogenesis. Furthermore, exogenous androgen administration is increasingly employed by amateur body builders, but profoundly impairs spermatogenesis.

Genetics of testicular failure

Genetic abnormalities [19] account for 10–15% of male factor infertility and can be broadly classified into chromosomal abnormalities, Y-chromosome microdeletions, X-linked gene mutations, autosomal gene mutations, polymorphisms and epigenetic errors.

Chromosomal abnormalities

The overall prevalence of chromosomal abnormalities is estimated to be around 5% in infertile men, but over 10% in azoospermic men [20]. The most common chromosome abnormality associated with male infertility is Klinefelter's syndrome caused by the 47,XXY karyotype (or 47,XXY/46,XY mosaics). Klinefelter's causes primary testicular failure during early adulthood, with increased gonadotrophins and low testosterone. It had previously been assumed that these patients had complete azoospermia, it has now been reported that approximately 25% may have evidence of spermatozoa on semen analysis although spontaneous conception is rare [21]. Recent reports suggest that microsurgical testicular sperm extraction (mTESE) followed by intracytoplasmic sperm injection (ICSI) could be used to successfully achieve conception in patients with Klinefelter's syndrome [22]; however it should be emphasised to patients that the chance of sperm retrieval is low and patients should be counselled regarding the increased risk of chromosome aneuploidy and the possibility of performing preimplantation genetic diagnosis (PGD). Another aneuploidy which can occur is 47,XYY syndrome which occurs in 1 in 1,000 live male births [23]. There is a higher prevalence in infertile men although many with this condition may be fertile. Patients may have a normal phenotype and testosterone level however tall stature, behavioural problems, delayed language skills and mild learning disability may feature. In contrast to Klinefelter's there does not appear to be an increased risk of aneuploidy in the offspring of patients with XYY. Men with azoospermia may rarely have a 46,XX karyotype [24]; a fragment of the Y-chromosome containing the *SRY* gene causes male sexual differentiation, but the absence of other genes on the Y-chromosome is incompatible with spermatogenesis. Chromosome translocations may also be associated with male infertility. Robertsonian translocations occur when two acrocentric chromosomes (13, 14, 15, 21, 22) fuse together. It has been reported that 0.8% of infertile men are carriers of a Robertsonian translocation which is up to nine times higher than the general population [25]. Reciprocal translocations involve an exchange of genetic material between two nonhomologous chromosomes. The incidence of reciprocal translocations has been reported to be seven times higher in infertile men than couples who have had a live birth [21]. Carriers of balanced translocations may have a normal phenotype however as there is a risk that children may inherit an unbalanced translocation these patients should also be offered genetic counselling. It is also possible to have X-autosomal and Y-autosomal translocations, the resulting impact on fertility is determined by the location of the breakpoints.

Y-chromosome microdeletions

The Y-chromosome contains genes which are crucial for male gonadal development and spermatogenesis. Microdeletions in the Yq11 region on the long arm of the Y-chromosome known as the azoospermic factor (AZF) region are prevalent in 10–15% of cases of non-obstructive azoospermia and 5–10% of severe oligozoospermia [26]. A microdeletion may span several genes. These are commonly subdivided into three regions. Deletions of the AZFa region have the worst prognosis for any Y-microdeletion, since they are largely incompatible with spermatogenesis. Deletions in the AZFb region also have a poor prognosis, with incomplete spermatogenesis and azoospermia. However, deletions of the AZFc may be compatible with a degree of spermatogenesis in some patients. AZFc microdeletions (including the *DAZ* gene family) are the most common type of Y microdeletion. It is important to note that affected patients with successful sperm retrieval should be given genetic counselling since the Y microdeletion will be inherited by male offspring.

Gene mutations

Approximately 2% of infertile men have mutations in the androgen receptor gene located on the long arm of the X chromosome [20]. The androgen receptor gene plays an important role in spermatogenesis and patients may be oligo or azoospermic. Infertility may be the only presenting symptom however mutations can also lead to androgen insensitivity syndrome and the neurodegenerative disorder Kennedy's syndrome. The ubiquitin specific protease 26 (*USP26*) gene and the transcription regulator factor gene *TAF7L* gene, which are located on the X-chromosome, are recognised for their role in spermatogenesis. Two small cohort case control studies have shown a significant correlation between mutations in these genes in men with non-obstructive azoospermia [28,29]. Approximately 5% of men with cryptorchidism have mutations in the *INSL3* gene [30] (insulin-like 3 on chromosome 19) and its receptor *LGR8* (relaxin/insulin-like family peptide receptor 2 on chromosome 13). *INSL3* is a peptide produced by Leydig cells which has a role in the transabdominal descent of the testes by acting on the gubernaculum. Mutations in the *INSL3* gene may also be present in testicular dysgenesis syndrome which can include cryptorchidism, hypospadias, testicular cancer and infertility.

Genetic polymorphisms

It is possible that polymorphisms in exon 1 of the androgen receptor (AR) gene [31,32], Y-chromosome haplogroups [33,34], the enzyme 5-methylenetetrahydrofolate reductase

(MTHFR C677T) [35,36], the enzyme human DNA polymerase Υ (POLG) [37], the *DAZL* (deleted in azoospermia-like) gene [38], the FSH receptor gene [39] and the oestrogen receptor (ER) genes [40] may contribute to male infertility. However, studies have produced conflicting results and have been limited by sample size and heterogeneous phenotypes. Furthermore it is possible that the clinical effects of polymorphisms are influenced by other genetic predispositions or environmental factors.

OBSTRUCTIVE AZOOSPERMIA

Approximately 40% of azoospemia cases arise from obstruction arising anywhere between the rete testis and the ejaculatory ducts [41]. There are a multitude of causes of obstructive azoospermia (OA) including congenital unilateral and bilateral absence of the vas deferens, trauma, infections (including prostatitis), epididymitis previous radiotherapy and surgery. A previous history of infant hernia repair and infant hydrocele surgery substantially increases the risk of OA. Furthermore, epididymitis is becoming a more common cause of OA due to sexually transmitted infections such as chlamydia. Up to 90% of patients with congenital bilateral absence of the vas deferens (CBAVD) have mutations in the cystic-fibrosis transmembrane conductance regulator (*CFTR*) gene located on chromosome 7 [42]. These patients may have intact spermatogenesis which can be retrieved surgically from the testes or epididymis, and later used for treatment with ICSI. Genetic counselling and PGD should be advised due to the increased risk of cystic fibrosis if the female partner also carries a *CFTR* mutation.

HYPOTHALAMO-PITUITARY DISEASE

Secondary hypogonadism – also termed hypogonadotrophic hypogonadism (HH) – is caused by hypothalamic or pituitary disease resulting in low testosterone and low LH and FSH secretion. Pituitary disease accounts for the majority of cases of secondary hypogonadism.

Hypothalamic failure may be due to congenital or acquired GnRH deficiency. Congenital GnRH deficiency (CGD) is a rare disorder characterised by the deficient production, secretion or action of GnRH resulting in low FSH, LH and testosterone with otherwise normal pituitary function [43]. Clinical features of CGD are incomplete or absent puberty and infertility which may or may not occur in association with other developmental abnormalities including cleft lip or palate, dental agenesis, hearing impairment, renal agenesis and skeletal abnormalities. CGD in association with anosmia or hyposmia is termed Kallmann syndrome which results from incomplete embryonic migration of GnRH synthesising neurones from the olfactory placode to the hypothalamus. Alternatively, GnRH neuronal function may be deficient but smell is intact (i.e. normosmic CGD). Over the last two decades, mutations in several genes have been identified to cause either normosmic CGD, Kallman syndrome, or both. These studies are ongoing and reveal an increasingly complex neurohumeral network termed the GnRH pulse generator including kisspeptin, neurokinin B, dynorphin and substance P which regulate the pulsatile release of GnRH from the hypothalamus [44,45]. Over 25 causal genes for CGD have been identified so far and studies suggest at least 20% of cases are oligogenic. Up to 22% of patients with CGD manage to regain sexual function [46]. Hypothalamic GnRH deficiency may also be acquired during obesity, chronic disease, opioid misuse and severe weight loss.

CLINICAL APPROACH TO THE INFERTILE MALE PATIENT

Significant points to discuss when taking the history include shaving, libido, early morning erections, undescended testes and onset of puberty [47]. Past medical history includes mumps, sexually transmitted infections (STI), previous malignancy, any systemic or chronic disease, and erectile or ejaculatory problems. A surgical history of orchidopexy suggests that the patient had undescended testes which may have reduced function. Medication history includes over the counter and recreational drugs and any additional supplements. Adverse lifestyle factors should also be elicited as discussed previously. Clinical examination may reveal secondary sexual characteristics and gynaecomastia [48]. The testes should be palpated to assess volume with a Prader orchidometer or ultrasound. Semen analysis should be performed for all patients following abstinence of a minimum of two and a maximum of 7 days. Current WHO reference ranges [4] represent the 5th centile of the general population: semen volume >1.5 mL; sperm concentration > 15 million per mL; total sperm number >39 million spermatozoa per ejaculate; total motility >40%; vitality, i.e. live spermatozoa >58%; sperm morphology >4%. Sperm autoantibodies may be detected using the mixed antibody reaction (MAR) test or immunobeads with a normal range of <50% binding; however NICE do not currently recommend these tests [49]. Hormonal analysis should include early morning serum testosterone, oestradiol, LH, FSH and prolactin. Sex hormone binding globulin may also be measured to calculate free androgen index. Genetic testing should be performed for all patients with azoospermia and include a karyotype and tests for Y-chromosome microdeletions and *CFTR* mutations. Scrotal ultrasound is not routinely undertaken to assess male infertility unless a specific urological abnormality is found.

TREATMENT OF MALE INFERTILITY

The treatment of male infertility can include medical and surgical management [50,51], assisted reproduction and the use of donor sperm. Prior to embarking upon treatment couples should be advised about their chance of spontaneous conception with expectant management. Couples should also be given information on lifestyle factors, future treatment options and the availability of support groups and counselling services [49].

MEDICAL TREATMENT OF MALE INFERTILITY AND HYPOGONADISM

Testosterone therapy

Testosterone replacement is routinely given for patients with hypogonadism who are not attempting to conceive [50] (as it may inhibit spermatogenesis via negative feedback). Testosterone maintains virilisation and increases libido, sexual function, muscle strength, fat free mass and bone density. Several testosterone preparations are available including injectable depot preparations, cutaneous gels and oral agents. Orally administered testosterone must be conjugated to minimise first-pass metabolism, but topical or injectable testosterone does not require conjugation for bioavailability.

Testosterone therapy stimulates prostatic growth, increases haematocrit and may increase the risk of thrombosis [51–53]. Careful consideration is therefore required when contemplating testosterone therapy for patients with a contraindication such as known prostate or breast cancer, erythrocytosis and severe cardiovascular disease. Men over 50 should be screened for prostate cancer with measurement of PSA and a digital rectal examination prior to initiating therapy. The haematocrit should also be measured prior to commencing testosterone, again within 6 months and then yearly. Serum testosterone should also be measured within 3 months of initiating treatment or changing the dose and every 6–12 months when a stable level is reached.

It is interesting to consider whether men require testosterone therapy in old age. Unlike women, men do not experience an abrupt reduction in gonadal function (sometimes termed andropause). However, testosterone actions do reduce with increasing age in men. The Baltimore Longitudinal Study of Ageing observed that free and total testosterone levels were reduced in men aged 60–69 years [54]. The Massachusetts Male Aging Study observed that free and bioavailable testosterone reduced at on average 2% annually [55]. The European Male Ageing Study (EMAS) proposed the minimum criteria for the identification of late onset hypogonadism (LOH), which entailed the presence of three sexual symptoms (decreased sexual interest and morning erections and erectile dysfunction) in combination with total serum testosterone below 11 nmol/L and free calculated testosterone below 220 [56]. Using these criteria, the EMAS investigators observed that only 2% of men aged 40–79 years had LOH. Furthermore, they observed that LOH was generally associated with a total serum testosterone below 8 nmol/L. Much debate surrounds the issue of testosterone supplementation in ageing men, but it appears appropriate to consider therapy in patients fulfilling the criteria for LOH. However, the decision to initiate therapy should always involve a discussion with the patient regarding the risks of therapy in the context of their premorbid history.

Induction of spermatogenesis with gonadotrophin injections

Patients with hypothalamic or pituitary dysfunction may benefit from gonadotrophin therapy when conception is desired. Human chorionic gonadotrophin (hCG) is a first line treatment for sperm induction in patients who have undergone pubertal development [57]. hCG mimics the biological activity of LH by stimulating Leydig cells in the testes to produce testosterone. This action results in a high local concentration of testosterone in the testes which may be sufficient to stimulate Sertoli cells and initiate spermatogenesis. hCG may be delivered by subcutaneous or intramuscular injection and the dose should be titrated with the aim of maintaining a normal serum testosterone level. A recent consensus statement on the treatment of congenital hypogonadotrophic hypogonadism [43] recommended that hCG should be the first-line therapy for patients with some pubertal development (testicular volume >4 mL) and no history of undescended testes. If a patient is still azoospermic following 6 months of treatment with hCG then a preparation containing FSH (such as menotrophin) may be used in conjunction with hCG. However, it has been suggested that patients with a testicular volume of <4 mL could benefit from an alternative treatment regime [58,59] commencing with unopposed FSH followed by hCG (or GnRH) to stimulate the proliferation of immature Sertoli and germ cells in male patients who lack the testicular development associated with puberty. Pulsatile GnRH is an alternative treatment for secondary hypogonadism specifically due to hypothalamic dysfunction, but is technically difficult to deliver and is unavailable in most countries including the UK. If spermatogenesis is successfully induced and sufficient numbers of viable sperm are sampled then sperm cryopreservation should be offered which commonly prevents the need to repeat therapy. In a minority of patients, gonadotrophin therapy may fail to induce significant spermatogenesis; such cases may benefit for consideration of surgical sperm retrieval [60,61].

Hormonal therapies to stimulate endogenous gonadotrophin secretion

It is controversial whether any medical therapies successfully increase fertility in men with idiopathic oligo/asthenozoospermia [62–64]. Drugs studied in this context include antioestrogens. For example clomifene and tamoxifen are selective oestrogen receptor modulators which inhibit the negative feedback of oestrogen. One recent meta-analysis [65] reported that clomifene and tamoxifen were associated with a statistically significant increase in pregnancy rates; however another study [66] reported that there is insufficient evidence to indicate that they are an effective empirical treatment. Aromatase inhibitors such as anastrozole have also been used to treat patients with male infertility by blocking the conversion of testosterone to oestrogen. Studies have reported improved semen parameters but again there is insufficient evidence to indicate that aromatase inhibitors are an effective empirical treatment [67,68]. There is insufficient evidence to conclude whether or not drugs boosting endogenous LH and FSH can treat men with idiopathic oligo/asthenozoospermia. More robust evidence is required before advocating the routine use of such therapies to treat men with infertility.

Kisspeptin

Recent studies have highlighted that the hypothalamic neuropeptide called kisspeptin is needed for endogenous GnRH function. Furthermore, inactivating mutations in the kisspeptin signalling pathway cause hypogonadotrophic hypogonadism [69]. Human studies suggest that peripheral, exogenous administration of kisspeptin stimulates gonadotrophin secretion safely and potently [70], thus implicating a potential novel therapeutic application. However, further studies are required before considering kisspeptin as a clinical therapy which has advantages over existing therapeutic approaches.

Surgical management of male infertility

Surgical techniques play a vital role in the management of obstructive infertility, and an emerging role in the management of testicular failure. Percutaneous epididymal sperm aspiration (PESA) or microsurgical epididymal sperm aspiration (MESA) are highly effective techniques for collecting sperm during obstructive azoospermia, since spermatogenesis is often intact in affected patients [60,61]. Surgical sperm retrieval may also be used to obtain sperm from men with non-obstructive azoospermia or severe oligoaesthenospermia, which is insufficient for assisted reproductive technologies (ART) such as ICSI. The technique of testicular sperm extraction (TESE) may have high associated rates of haematoma and testicular devascularisation [71]. Therefore, microdissection TESE (mTESE) was introduced in 1999, which is now considered the gold-standard surgical procedure for surgical sperm retrieval. mTESE allows the microdissection and identification of individual tubules appearing to be engorged with spermatogenesis in situ (**Figure 7.2**) [72]. During mTESE, tubules are dissected by the surgeon and examined intraoperatively for sperm by an assistant. Samples are then sent to an andrological laboratory to cryopreserve sperm for ART. Sperm retrieval rates up to 60% may be observed with mTESE in specialist centres, although results will vary on patient characteristics and surgical experience [73].

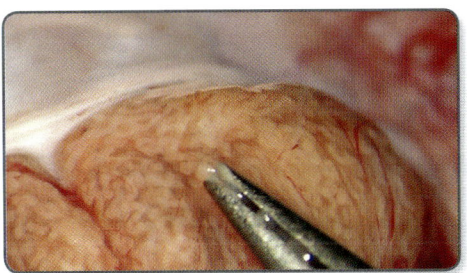

Figure 7.2 Intra-operative image from microdissection testicular sperm retrieval (mTESE). A single seminiferous tubule is held using micro-forceps prior to dissection, microscopic examination for sperm, and processing prior to sperm cryopreservation.

CONCLUSION

Male infertility is common and has devastating consequences for patients. Several recent advances have highlighted emerging roles for lifestyle factors and genetics in the pathogenesis of male infertility. However, treatment options for male infertility remain limited, unless gonadotrophin therapy is administered for patients with hypothalamo-pituitary dysfunction. Further advances in therapeutics of male infertility are required to reduce reliance on ART such as ICSI and donor sperm. Testosterone therapy should be considered in patients with hypogonadism associated with sexual symptoms; however, the benefits of therapy should outweigh the risk of potential complications for the individual patient.

Key points for clinical practice

- Investigation of the infertile male should include semen analysis. In 2010 the WHO published revised reference ranges for semen analysis. These values represent the 5th centile of the general population: Semen volume > 1.5 mL; sperm concentration > 15 million per mL, total sperm number > 39 million spermatozoa per ejaculate, total motility > 40%, vitality, i.e. live spermatozoa > 58%, sperm morphology > 4%. Investigations should also include hormonal analysis (including early morning serum testosterone, oestradiol, LH, FSH and prolactin. Sex hormone binding globulin may also be measured to calculate the free androgen index) and genetic testing for all patients with azoospermia (including a karyotpye, Y-chromosome microdeletions and CFTR mutations). Genetic counselling and PGD should be offered if required.

- Patients should be counselled on lifestyle factors including obesity, alcohol intake and smoking.

- Medical management of male infertility may be successful for patients with hypogonadotrophic hypogonadism. hCG is the first line treatment for sperm induction in patients who have undergone pubertal development. There is not yet any evidence-based empirical treatment for idiopathic oligo/asthenozoospermia. Testosterone therapy is not a suitable treatment for patients attempting to conceive.

- Surgical sperm retrieval may be successful for patients with obstructive male infertility and in some cases severe oligo or azoospermia including in the context of Klinefelter's syndrome. Microsurgical testicular sperm extraction (mTESE) is now the gold standard technique and the aim is to facilitate assisted reproduction treatment with ICSI.

REFERENCES

1. Zegers-Hochschild F, Adamson GD, de Mouzon J, et al. International Committee for Monitoring Assisted Reproductive Technology (ICMART) and the World Health Organization (WHO) revised glossary of ART terminology. Fertil Steril 2009; 92:1520–1524.
2. te Velde ER, Eijkemans R, Habbema HD. Variation in couple fecundity and time to pregnancy, an essential concept in human reproduction. Lancet 2000; 355:1928–9.
3. Human Fertilisation and Embryology Authority. Success rates - IVF Hammersmith. London: Human Fertilisation and Embryology Authority; 2015.
4. World Health Organization, Department of Reproductive Health and Research. WHO laboratory manual for the examination and processing of human semen. Geneva: World Health Organization; 2010.
5. Johnson MH. Essential Reproduction. 6th Ed. London: Wiley-Blackwell; 2007.
6. Misell LM, Holochwost D, Boban D, et al. A stable isotope-mass spectrometric method for measuring human spermatogenesis kinetics in vivo. J Urol 2006; 175:242–246.
7. Karavolos S, Stewart J, Evbuomwan I, McEleny K, Aird I. Assessment of the infertile male. Obstet Gynaecol 2013; 15:1–9.
8. Esteves SC, Hamada A, Kondray V, Pitchika A, Agarwal A. What every gynecologist should know about male infertility: an update. Arch Gynecol Obstet 2012; 286:217–229.
9. Stahl PJ, Stember DS, Goldstein M. Contemporary management of male infertility. Annu Rev Med 2012; 63:525–540.
10. Krausz C. Male infertility: pathogenesis and clinical diagnosis. Best Pract Res Clin Endocrinol Metab 2011; 25:271–285.
11. Agarwal A, Hamada A, Esteves SC. Engaging practicing gynecologists in the management of infertile men. J Obstet Gynaecol India 2015; 65:75–87.
12. Brezina PR, Yunus FN, Zhao Y. Effects of pharmaceutical medications on male fertility. J Reprod Infertil 2012; 13:3–11.
13. Nudell DM, Monoski MM, Lipshultz LI. Common medications and drugs: how they affect male fertility. Urol Clin North Am 2002; 29:965–973.
14. Du Plessis SS, Cabler S, McAlister DA, Sabanegh E, Agarwal A. The effect of obesity on sperm disorders and male infertility. Nat Rev Urol 2010; 7:153–161.
15. Luboshitzky R, Lavie L, Shen-Orr Z, Herer P. Altered luteinizing hormone and testosterone secretion in middle-aged obese men with obstructive sleep apnea. Obes Res 2005; 13:780–786.
16. Alshahrani S, Ahmed AF, Gabr AH, Abalhassan M, Ahmad G. The impact of body mass index on semen parameters in infertile men. Andrologia 2016.
17. Muthusami KR, Chinnaswamy P. Effect of chronic alcoholism on male fertility hormones and semen quality. Fertil Steril 2005; 84:919–924.
18. Practice Committee of the American Society for Reproductive Medicine. Smoking and infertility: a committee opinion. Fertil Steril 2012; 98:1400–1406.
19. O'Flynn O'Brien KL, Varghese AC, Agarwal A. The genetic causes of male factor infertility: A review. Fertil Steril 2010; 93:1–12.
20. Foresta C, Ferlin A, Gianaroli L, Dallapiccola B. Guidelines for the appropriate use of genetic tests in infertile couples. Eur J Hum Genet 2002; 10:303–312.
21. Ferlin A, Raicu F, Gatta V, Zuccarello D, Palka G, Foresta C. Male infertility: role of genetic background. Reprod Biomed Online 2007; 14:734–745.
22. Ramasamy R, Ricci JA, Palermo GD, Gosden LV, Rosenwaks Z, Schlegel PN. Successful fertility treatment for Klinefelter's syndrome. J Urol 2009; 182:1108–1113.
23. Kim IW, Khadilkar AC, Ko EY, Sabanegh ES. 47,XYY syndrome and male infertility. Rev Urol 2013;15:188–196.
24. Ryan NAJ, Akbar S. A case report of an incidental finding of a 46,XX, SRY-negative male with masculine phenotype during standard fertility workup with review of the literature and proposed immediate and long-term management guidance. Fertil Steril 2013; 99:1273–1276.
25. De Braekeleer M, Dao TN. Cytogenetic studies in male infertility: a review. Hum Reprod 1991; 6:245–250.
26. Foresta C, Moro E, Ferlin A. Y chromosome microdeletions and alterations of spermatogenesis. Endocr Rev 2001; 22:226–239.
27. Ferlin A, Vinanzi C, Garolla A, Selice R, Zuccarello D, Cazzadore C, et al. Male infertility and androgen receptor gene mutations: clinical features and identification of seven novel mutations. Clin Endocrinol (Oxf) 2006; 65:606–610.

28. Paduch DA, Mielnik A, Schlegel PN. Novel mutations in testis-specific ubiquitin protease 26 gene may cause male infertility and hypogonadism. Reprod Biomed Online 2005; 10:747–754.

29. Akinloye O, Gromoll J, Callies C, Nieschlag E, Simoni M. Mutation analysis of the X-chromosome linked, testis-specific TAF7L gene in spermatogenic failure. Andrologia 2007; 39:190–195.

30. Ferlin A, Foresta C. Insulin-like factor 3: a novel circulating hormone of testicular origin in humans. Ann NY Acad Sci 2005; 1041:497–505.

31. Tut TG, Ghadessy FJ, Trifiro MA, Pinsky L, Yong EL. Long polyglutamine tracts in the androgen receptor are associated with reduced trans-activation, impaired sperm production, and male infertility. J Clin Endocrinol Metab 1997; 82:3777–3782.

32. Lazaros L, Xita N, Kaponis A, Zikopoulos K, Sofikitis N, Georgiou I. Evidence for association of sex hormone-binding globulin and androgen receptor genes with semen quality. Andrologia 2008; 40:186–191.

33. Arredi B, Ferlin A, Speltra E, et al. Y-chromosome haplogroups and susceptibility to azoospermia factor c microdeletion in an Italian population. J Med Genet 2007; 44:205–208.

34. Repping S, Skaletsky H, Brown L, et al. Polymorphism for a 1.6-Mb deletion of the human Y chromosome persists through balance between recurrent mutation and haploid selection. Nat Genet 2003; 35:247–251.

35. Park JH, Lee HC, Jeong Y-M, et al. MTHFR C677T polymorphism associates with unexplained infertile male factors. J Assist Reprod Genet 2005; 22:361–368.

36. Singh K, Singh SK, Sah R, Singh I, Raman R. Mutation C677T in the methylenetetrahydrofolate reductase gene is associated with male infertility in an Indian population. Int J Androl 2005; 28:115–119.

37. Rovio AT, Marchington DR, Donat S, et al. Mutations at the mitochondrial DNA polymerase (POLG) locus associated with male infertility. Nat Genet 2005; 29:261–262.

38. Tung JY, Rosen MP, Nelson LM, et al. Novel missense mutations of the Deleted-in-AZoospermia-Like (DAZL) gene in infertile women and men. Reprod Biol Endocrinol 2006; 4:40.

39. Ahda Y, Gromoll J, Wunsch A, et al. Follicle-stimulating hormone receptor gene haplotype distribution in normozoospermic and azoospermic men. J Androl 2005; 26:494–499.

40. Guarducci E, Nuti F, Becherini L, et al. Estrogen receptor alpha promoter polymorphism: stronger estrogen action is coupled with lower sperm count. Hum Reprod 2006; 21:994–1001.

41. Wosnitzer M, Goldstein M, Hardy MP. Review of azoospermia. Spermatogenesis 2014; 4:e28218.

42. Georgiou I, Syrrou M, Pardalidis N, et al. Genetic and epigenetic risks of intracytoplasmic sperm injection method. Asian J Androl 2006; 8:643–673.

43. Boehm U, Bouloux P-M, Dattani MT, et al. Expert consensus document: European Consensus Statement on congenital hypogonadotropic hypogonadism – pathogenesis, diagnosis and treatment. Nat Rev Endocrinol 2015; 11:547–564.

44. Hameed S, Jayasena CN, Dhillo WS. Kisspeptin and fertility. J Endocrinol 2011; 208:97–105.

45. Clarke H, Dhillo WS, Jayasena CN. Comprehensive review on kisspeptin and its role in reproductive disorders. Endocrinol Metab (Seoul, Korea) 2015; 30:124–141.

46. Sidhoum VF, Chan Y-M, Lippincott MF, Balasubramanian R, Quinton R, Plummer L, et al. Reversal and relapse of hypogonadotropic hypogonadism: resilience and fragility of the reproductive neuroendocrine system. J Clin Endocrinol Metab 2014; 99:861–870.

47. Reynard J, Brewster S, Biers S. Oxford Handbook of Urology. 3rd ed. Oxford: Oxford University Press; 2013.

48. Reynard , Mark S, Turner K, et al. Oxford Specialist Handbook of Urological Surgery. Oxford: Oxford University Press; 2008.

49. National Institute for Health and Care Excellence. Fertility problems: assessment and treatment. Manchester: National Institute for Health and Care Excellence; 2013.

50. Miner M, Barkin J, Rosenberg MT. Testosterone deficiency: myth, facts, and controversy. Can J Urol 2014; 21:39–54.

51. Fowler JE, Whitmore WF. The response to metastatic adenocarcinoma of the prostate to exogenous testosterone. J Urol 1981; 126: 372–375.

52. Jacobsen SJ, Girman CJ, Lieber MM. Natural history of benign prostatic hyperplasia. Urology 2001; 58:5–16.

53. Krauss DJ, Taub HA, Lantinga LJ, Dunsky MH, Kelly CM. Risks of blood volume changes in hypogonadal men treated with testosterone enanthate for erectile impotence. J Urol 1991; 146:1566–1570.

54. Harman SM, Metter EJ, Tobin JD, Pearson J, Blackman MR. Longitudinal effects of aging serum total and free testosterone levels in healthy men. Baltimore Longitudinal Study of Aging. J Clin Endocrinol Metab 2001; 86:724–731.

55. Feldman HA, Longscope C, Derby CA, et al. Age trends in the level of serum testosterone and other hormones in middle aged men: longitudional results from the Massachusettes Male Aging Study. J Clin Endocrinol Metab 2002; 87:589–598.

56. Tajar A, Huhthaiemi LT, O'Neill JD, et al. Characteristcs of androgen deficiency in late-onset hypogonadism: results from the European Male Aging Study (EMAS). J Clin Endocrinol Metab 2012; 97:1509–1516.

57. Imperial College Healthcare NHS Trust. Fertility induction in hypogonadotrophic hypogonadism. In: Endocrinology Handbook. London: Imperial College Healthcare NHS Trust, 1988.

58. Dwyer AA, Sykiotis GP, Hayes FJ, et al. Trial of recombinant follicle-stimulating hormone pretreatment for GnRH-induced fertility in patients with congenital hypogonadotropic hypogonadism. J Clin Endocrinol Metab 2013; 98:E1790–E1795.

59. Raivio T, Wikström AM, Dunkel L. Treatment of gonadotropin-deficient boys with recombinant human FSH: long-term observation and outcome. Eur J Endocrinol 2007; 156:105–111.

60. Dabaja AA, Schlegel PN. Microdissection testicular sperm extraction: an update. Asian J Androl 2013; 15:35–39.

61. Shin DH, Turek PJ. Sperm retrieval techniques. Nat Rev Urol 2013; 10:723–730.

62. Garg H, Kumar R. Empirical drug therapy for idiopathic male infertility: what is the new evidence? Urology 2915; 86:1065–1075.

63. Jung JH, Seo JT. Empirical medical therapy in idiopathic male infertility: promise or panacea? Clin Exp Reprod Med 2014; 41:108–114.

64. Rittenberg V, El-Toukhy T. Medical treatment of male infertility. Hum Fertil (Camb) 2010; 13:208–216.

65. Chua ME, Escusa KG, Luna S, et al. Revisiting oestrogen antagonists (clomiphene or tamoxifen) as medical empiric therapy for idiopathic male infertility: a meta-analysis. Andrology 2013; 1:749–757.

66. Willets AE, Corbo JM, Brown JN. Clomiphene for the treatment of male infertility. Reprod Sci 2013; 20:739–744.

67. Schlegel PN. Aromatase inhibitors for male infertility. Fertil Steril 2012; 98:1359–1362.

68. Liu PY, Handelsman DJ. The present and future state of hormonal treatment for male infertility. Hum Reprod Update 2015; 9:9–23.

69. Seminara SB, Messager S, Chatzidaki EE, et al. The GPR54 gene as a regulator of puberty. N Engl J Med 2003; 349:1614–1627.

70. Jayasena CN, Abbara A, Narayanaswamy S, et al. Direct comparison of the effects of intravenous kisspeptin-10, kisspeptin-54 and GnRH on gonadotrophin secretion in healthy men. Hum Reprod 2015; 30:1934–1941.

71. Deruyve Y, Vanderschueren D, Van der Aa F. Outcome of microdissection TESE compared with conventional TESE in non-obstructive azoospermia: a systematic review. Andrology 2014; 2:20–24.

72. Ramasamy R, Lin K ,Godsen LV, et al. High serum FSH levels in men with non obstructive azoopsermia does not affect success of microdissection testicular sperm extraction. Fertil Steril 2009; 92:590–593.

73. Inci K, Hascicek M, Kara O, et al. Sperm retrieval and intracytoplasmic sperm injection in men with non-obstructive azoopsermia and treated and untreated varicocele. J Urol 2009; 182:1500–1505.

Chapter 8

Kisspeptin: a multifunctional hormone with emerging roles

Waljit Dhillo, Chioma Izzi-Engbeaya

INTRODUCTION

The kisspeptins are encoded by the *KISS1* gene, which is found on chromosome 1 [1]. *KISS1* was discovered in 1996 and it produces a 145-amino-acid peptide, which is enzymatically broken down into shorter peptides. These shorter peptides are kisspeptins with a numerical suffix added to indicate the length of their amino acid chains. The smallest kisspeptin is kisspeptin-10, which consists of a 10-amino-acid C-terminal chain that is found in all kisspeptins and is essential for their biological activity [2]. In humans, the kisspeptin predominantly produced from the precursor peptide is kisspeptin-54 (previously known as metastin), but other kisspeptins found in the circulation include kisspeptin-13 and kisspeptin-14 [3].

Kisspeptin-producing neurones are found in the infundibular nucleus [4] and preoptic area of the hypothalamus [5], as well as the amygdala [6]. Kisspeptin is also produced by pituitary gonadotrophs [6], the placenta [6], testis [3], ovary [7,8], uterus [9], pancreas [3], small intestine [3] and the adrenal glands [10]. Kisspeptin activates the G-protein coupled receptor called the kisspeptin receptor (KISS1R, which is also known as GPR54). This receptor is found in the hypothalamus [6,11], amygdala [6,11], anterior pituitary [6], cerebral cortex [6,11], cerebellum [6], placenta [3,6], testis [3], ovary [7,8], uterus [9], pancreas [3,6], liver [11] and adrenal glands [12].

Initial reports were focused on the ability of kisspeptin-54 to suppress metastasis of certain types of cancer [1]. More recently there has been a rapid expansion in the research into and subsequent knowledge of the pivotal roles kisspeptin plays in reproduction. Additionally, it is becoming apparent that kisspeptin may affect other important biological systems. In this chapter, current knowledge of kisspeptin's actions in humans will be summarised and the potential uses of kisspeptin signalling in the development of therapeutic agents will be discussed.

Waljit Dhillo BSc MBBS PhD FRCP FRCPath, Department of Endocrinology & Diabetes, Hammersmith Hospital, London, UK. Email: w.dhillo@imperial.ac.uk (for correspondence).

Chioma Izzi-Engbeaya BSc MBBS MRCP, Section of Investigative Medicine, Imperial College London, London, UK.

KISSPEPTIN AND REPRODUCTION

Currently, most of the published literature has focused on kisspeptin's roles in reproduction. Therefore, there is more knowledge about this aspect of kisspeptin function than any other functions of kisspeptin. The various aspects of kisspeptin's functions in reproduction, with an emphasis on human studies, are described below.

Regulation of reproductive hormones

Electron microscopy has revealed that kisspeptin fibres make direct contact with gonadotrophin releasing hormone (GnRH) neurones [13]. Most GnRH neurones express KISS1R [14], and kisspeptin acts directly on GnRH neurones to stimulate GnRH secretion [15-17]. Central (in animals) [15,16] and peripheral (animals and humans) [15,18] administration of kisspeptin results in an increase in circulating luteinising hormone (LH) and follicle stimulating hormone (FSH) levels. Kisspeptin administration does not cause a rise in gonadotrophins when the hypothalamus has been disconnected from the pituitary [19] or when a GnRH antagonist is administered prior to kisspeptin administration [14]. Therefore, it is likely that kisspeptin causes gonadotrophin secretion indirectly via its ability to stimulate GnRH secretion. However, kisspeptin may have a direct (albeit minor) effect on pituitary gonadotropes as these cells express *KISS1* [6] and KISS1R [19], and when pituitary tissue explants are exposed to kisspeptin, there is a dose-dependent increase in LH [19]. Interestingly, neither acute nor chronic subcutaneous kisspeptin-54 administration produces increases in serum prolactin, thyroid stimulating hormone and growth hormone levels (with the frequency and amplitude of growth hormone levels remaining unchanged) [20]. Therefore, kisspeptin specifically increases gonadotrophins but no other anterior pituitary hormones.

Kisspeptin is likely to be involved in the feedback of sex steroids on gonadotrophin secretion. Sex steroids (oestrogen, testosterone and dihydrotestosterone) inhibit kisspeptin expression in the arcuate nucleus [21,22], but they increase kisspeptin expression in the anteroventral periventricular nucleus (the rodent homologue of the human preoptic area) [21,22]. Kisspeptin-10 administration stimulates LH secretion in women in the follicular phase of the menstrual cycle and in post-menopausal (i.e. oestrogen-deficient) women but not in women taking oestrogen-containing contraceptive pills, and the greatest increase in LH levels are seen in post-menopausal women [23]. In females, oestrogen exerts a negative feedback effect on gonadotrophin secretion throughout the menstrual cycle apart from mid-cycle when it exerts a positive feedback effect, which produces the pre-ovulatory surge in LH that is crucial for fertility. The oestrogen receptor (ER) exists in two isoforms, ERα and ERβ, and signalling via ERα (but not via ERβ) is essential for the positive feedback effect of oestrogen [24]. Kisspeptin neurones express both isoforms of the ER and the androgen receptor [21,22], whilst GnRH neurones express ERβ but not ERα [25,26]. Female rodents treated with an ERα antagonist have a reduced response to kisspeptin-10 and they do not experience a pre-ovulatory LH peak nor do they ovulate [27]. Further work is required to fully elucidate kisspeptin's roles within these positive and negative feedback mechanisms.

Puberty

Puberty is triggered by the activation of the hypothalamus–pituitary–gonadal axis with the onset of regular pulses of GnRH, which causes pulsatile gonadotrophin and sex hormone secretion and resultant maturation of the reproductive system. Kisspeptin-expressing neurones [28], kisspeptin-GnRH neurone connections [29], frequency of kisspeptin pulses [30], hypothalamic kisspeptin mRNA expression [31] and kisspeptin receptor sensitivity [31] increase postpubertally compared with prepubertally. Activating mutations of *KISS1* [32] or *KISS1R* [33] cause precocious puberty, while higher kisspeptin levels than age-matched controls are found in children with precocious puberty who are not known to have these activating mutations [34]. Furthermore, plasma levels of kisspeptin are higher in children (aged 1–17) compared with adults (aged ≥ 19), with peak kisspeptin levels occurring in the 9–12 years (i.e. peripubertal) age group [35]. Individuals with inactivating mutations of *KISS1* [36] or *KISS1R* [37–39] have hypogonadotrophic hypogonadism and spontaneous pubertal development does not occur. Therefore, normal kisspeptin release and action is required for appropriate pubertal timing, initiation and progression.

Men

Kisspeptin was first administered to human volunteers in 2005 by Dhillo et al., and in this study a 4-hour infusion of kisspeptin 54 resulted in increases in LH, FSH and testosterone with the largest increases seen in LH [18]. Both a single bolus of kisspeptin-10 and intravenous infusions of kisspeptin-10 produce dose-dependent increases in serum LH concentrations, but tachyphylaxis occurs at higher doses [40,41]. Compared to endogenous LH pulses, exogenous kisspeptin-10 stimulated LH pulses have larger amplitudes and last longer [42]. Intravenous kisspeptin-10 infusions also increase LH pulse frequency [40]. In contrast, a single bolus of kisspeptin-10 delays the appearance of the subsequent endogenous LH pulse, and thus kisspeptin may have the ability to reset the GnRH pulse generator in men [42].

Kisspeptin-10 administration also increases serum testosterone levels [40,41]. Bolus intravenous kisspeptin-10 increases serum LH to the same extent in men with type 2 diabetes with asymptomatic biochemically low testosterone levels as nondiabetic men with normal testosterone levels, and kisspeptin-10 infusion increases the LH pulse frequency in this group of men with type 2 diabetes [43]. GnRH, kisspeptin-10 and kisspeptin-54 increase gonadotrophin levels compared to baseline and placebo in healthy men, however intravenous GnRH infusions produce 3-fold higher levels of LH and FSH than equimolar kisspeptin-10 infusions and 2-fold higher LH and FSH levels than equimolar kisspeptin-54 infusions [44]. Further work is required to fully characterise the role kisspeptin plays in the human male reproductive system.

Women

The female reproductive system has to be flexible enough to ensure that regular menstrual cycles occur and adapt to facilitate pregnancy and lactation. The studies outlined below have shed some light on the roles kisspeptin plays in various physiological and pathological states in females.

Healthy women with regular cycles

As discussed above, kisspeptin signalling appears to be essential for the positive and negative feedback of oestrogens on gonadotrophin secretion, which is required for menstrual cyclicity and the mid-cycle LH surge that causes ovulation. Intravenous kisspeptin-10 increases LH in women in the follicular phase of their cycles in some studies [23], but not in others [41]. Acute and/or chronic intravenous and/or subcutaneous kisspeptin-54 increases LH levels in women in all phases of the menstrual cycle [45,46].

The effect of kisspeptin-54 is most potent in the preovulatory phase (which has higher oestrogen levels) and least potent in the follicular phase (which has lower oestrogen levels) [45]. Furthermore, the magnitude of the acute increase in LH during subcutaneous infusion of kisspeptin-54 in the follicular phase is positively correlated with the baseline oestrogen levels [47]. Not only does kisspeptin play a role in the control of gonadotrophin release, it can influence the length of the menstrual cycle as chronic kisspeptin-54 administration for 7 days during the follicular phase of the cycle shortens the length of the menstrual cycle by 2 days [46].

Pregnancy

In pregnancy, kisspeptin is produced by the brain and placenta. Circulating kisspeptin levels are at least 100–1000 times higher in pregnant women compared to non-pregnant women (and men) [48,49]. Unlike human chorionic gonadotrophin (hCG) which peaks around the 8th gestational week, kisspeptin levels continue to increase throughout pregnancy [49,50]. Elevated kisspeptin immunoreactivity is found in the urine of pregnant women in the third trimester compared to non-pregnant women [48]. Among pregnant women, lower kisspeptin levels in early pregnancy are found in obese women [51], women with pre-existing type 1 diabetes or hypertension [52], and in those who subsequently develop pre-eclampsia [51,53], are asymptomatic at the time of the blood test but subsequently miscarry [50], and in women who experience bleeding between 7 and 18 weeks and have antenatal complications [54]. First trimester kisspeptin levels increase with the number of living fetuses, but the loss of one fetus in twin pregnancies results in similar kisspeptin levels to those found in singleton pregnancies [50]. Third trimester kisspeptin levels are lower in women whose pregnancies are complicated by pre-eclampsia or gestational diabetes [52]. In women with pre-eclampsia, lower kisspeptin levels are found in those with abnormal uterine artery Doppler velocities and kisspeptin levels are inversely correlated with proteinuria [55].

Carefully regulated placental invasion of the maternal uterus is necessary for the survival of the implanted embryo and developing fetus, and accumulating evidence suggests that kisspeptin is involved in the regulation of placental invasion. The placental expression of kisspeptin and its receptor in normal pregnancies is higher in early pregnancy (7–9 weeks) when the placenta is more invasive compared with late pregnancy (39–41 weeks) when the placenta is less invasive [56]. Kisspeptin-10 inhibits the migration of placental tissue [57] possibly by increasing adhesion of trophoblastic cells to type-1 collagen within the placental matrix [58]. Furthermore kisspeptin-10 has a concentration-dependent inhibitory effect on placental artery angiogenesis [59].

Lower placental *KISS1* [60] and KISS1R expression in early pregnancy are associated with recurrent spontaneous miscarriage [61]. At term, higher KISS1R expression [62], and both lower [62] and higher [63,64] *KISS1* expression have been found in placentas from pre-eclampsia pregnancies following caesarean section. Hopefully, as further research is performed, the roles kisspeptin plays in pregnancy and its usefulness as a marker of pregnancies at increased risk of complications will become clearer.

Hyperprolactinaemia (physiological and pathological)

Interactions between kisspeptin and prolactin neurones might be a mechanism by which hyperprolactinaemia causes reduced LH and FSH secretion. Most kisspeptin neurones have prolactin receptors (while only 5% of GnRH neurons have prolactin receptors) [65] and prolactin administration acts directly on kisspeptin neurones to inhibit kisspeptin expression and indirectly reduce LH secretion in mice [66] and rats [67]. Lactating rats have endogenously high prolactin levels with low kisspeptin expression in the arcuate nucleus and low plasma LH, which is partly reversed by central or peripheral bromocriptine administration [67]. Additionally, in female mice in which hyperprolactinaemia was produced by a continuous subcutaneous prolactin infusion, reduced hypothalamic kisspeptin expression, unchanged GnRH expression but reduced GnRH release, reduced LH expression (with reduced circulating LH and FSH levels) and loss of ovarian cyclicity occurred [68]. Daily intraperitoneal kisspeptin injections given to these hyperprolactinaemic mice restored GnRH levels, reversed the suppression of LH and FSH levels and restored ovarian cycles [68].

Rodent studies have shown that central administration of high doses of kisspeptin-10 stimulates prolactin secretion via inhibition of dopamine-secreting neurones and this effect is dependent on oestrogen [69,70]. In contrast, intravenous administration of kisspeptin-10 to male monkeys does not increase circulating prolactin levels [71], and peripheral administration of kisspeptin-54 to healthy women with regular menstrual cycles (at doses that result in significant elevations in gonadotrophins) acutely and twice daily subcutaneously for 7 days produces prolactin levels that are no different from those measured after vehicle administration [20]. These contrasting results indicate that the relationship between exogenous kisspeptin administration and prolactin secretion may be dependent on the route of administration and the species studied and this has to be taken into account whilst interpreting these studies.

Functinal hypothalamic amenorrhea

Functional hypothalamic amenorrhea (FHA) is hypogonadotrophic hypogonadism with resultant secondary amenorrhea in otherwise healthy women with normal neuroanatomy and pubertal development. Common causes include stress, excessive physical activity and weight loss/low body weight [72]. Subcutaneous injection of kisspeptin-54 acutely stimulates gonadotrophin secretion in women with FHA [73], and 8-hour intravenous infusions of kisspeptin-54 increase LH pulsatility in these women [74]. In FHA almost complete desensitisation occurs when kisspeptin-54 (6.4 nmol/kg) is administered subcutaneously twice daily for 2 weeks [73], but the gonadotrophin response to kisspeptin is partially preserved if kisspeptin-54 (6.4 nmol/kg) is administered subcutaneously twice weekly for 8 weeks [75]. During 8-hour kisspeptin-54 infusions there is a dose-dependent increase in gonadotrophin levels, but desensitisation occurs after 5 hours of infusion at doses exceeding 0.3 nmol/kg/h [74]. Furthermore this desensitisation does not appear to occur at the level of the pituitary because identical responses to GnRH are obtained immediately following the cessation of the 1 nmol/kg/h infusion and 7 days after the infusion was stopped [74].

Leptin-kisspeptin interaction may explain why FHA can occur after excess weight loss and/or in women with low body weight. Leptin is an anorectic hormone produced by adipocytes in quantities that are proportional to body fat, and it informs the brain of the body's energy stores [76–78]. Fasting reduces leptin levels and refeeding increases leptin levels in humans [79]. Kisspeptin neurones express the leptin receptor [80] but GnRH neurones do not express the leptin receptor [81]. Ob/ob mice are leptin-deficient, have hypogonadotrophic hypogonadism [82], have low kisspeptin levels, whilst kisspeptin levels increase [80] and infertility is reversed by the administration of leptin [83]. Similarly, people with congenital leptin deficiency have hypogonadotrophic hypogonadism [84], and leptin treatment enables puberty to occur [85]. In FHA, not only are leptin levels low, the diurnal rhythm of leptin secretion is lost [86]. Administration of recombinant leptin to women with FHA restores LH pulsatility (with the resumption of ovulatory menstrual cycles in some women) [87]. Further work is required to fully elucidate the kisspeptin-leptin relationship in FHA.

Postmenopausal women/women with premature ovarian failure

Following ovarian failure (either premature or menopausal), oestrogen levels are very low and gonadotrophin levels are markedly elevated. In the hypothalami of postmenopausal women, there are a greater number of kisspeptin-expressing neurones and these neurones are bigger in size and express double the amount of KISS1 mRNA compared to premenopausal women [4]. However, no significant differences in circulating kisspeptin levels have been found in postmenopausal women/women with premature ovarian failure (POF) compared with women with regular menstrual cycles [88,89]. Postmenopausal women retain the ability to increase gonadotrophin secretion in response to kisspeptin-10 and are more sensitive to kisspeptin-10 than premenopausal women in the follicular phase of the menstrual cycle (likely due to their oestrogen-deficient state) [23].

Certain populations of kisspeptin neurons co-express a vasoactive peptide called neurokinin B (NKB) and dynorphin (collectively called KNDy neurones) [90]. These KNDy neurones are part of the pathway by which oestrogen suppresses gonadotrophin secretion via negative feedback [91] and may also be involved in the mechanism by which oestrogen deficiency (in menopause/POF) causes hot flushes [92].

KISSPEPTIN AND CANCER

In malignant melanoma [1] and breast [93] cancer, KISS1 expression is associated with greatly reduced metastatic potential. Conversely reduced KISS1 (or KISS1R) expression within cancer cells is associated with greater tumour invasion, metastasis and/or worse prognosis in uveal melanoma [94], gastric [95], oesophageal [96], gallbladder adenocarcinoma [97], bladder [98], breast [99], pancreatic [100], lung [101], renal cell [102], colorectal [103], nasopharyngeal [104], and ovarian [105,106] cancer. However, in hepatocellular [107,108], colorectal [109,110] and breast [111] cancer, higher KISS1 expression is associated with tumour progression and a worse clinical outcome, and in breast cancer this may be due to differences in ER status of breast tumours and oestrogen levels (premenopausal versus postmenopausal) of the affected women [112]. Therefore, the role of kisspeptin in tumour metastases and cancer progression remains controversial.

The mechanisms by which kisspeptin may reduce metastatic potential have not been fully characterised. However studies using human cancer cells lines and cancer tissue have shown that KISS1 expression reduces cell migration in pancreatic [113], ovarian [114] and renal cell [115] cancer cells, reduces proliferation and invasion of gastric cancer cells [116], and reduces invasiveness of prostate cancer [117] and osteosarcoma [118] cells. Kisspeptin-10 reduces cell proliferation and increases apoptosis in breast cancer cells [119], inhibits tumour angiogenesis [120], decreases migration of colorectal cancer cells [121], and inhibits invasion of endometrial cancer cells [122]. A lot more work remains to be done in this important field of study.

KISSPEPTIN AND THE CARDIOVASCULAR SYSTEM

In humans *KISS1* and KISS1R are expressed in the heart, coronary vessels and aorta, with lower kisspeptin levels found in the right atria of hearts from patients with ischaemic heart disease [123,124]. Both kisspeptin-10 and kisspeptin-54 have dose-dependent positive inotropic effects on strips of the atrial appendage [123] and act as vasoconstrictors in isolated coronary artery rings [124]. Kisspeptin-54 also increases aldosterone production in adrenal cells [12]. However, no increase in heart rate or blood pressure was detected in healthy male volunteers who received 90 minute infusions of kisspeptin-54 at doses ranging from 0–2.4 pmol/kg/min and healthy female volunteers who received subcutaneous boluses of kisspeptin-54 at doses of 0–6.4 nmol/kg [125]. Furthermore there is no positive correlation between plasma kisspeptin concentrations and either systolic or diastolic blood pressures in normotensive pregnant women, as well as women with pre-eclampsia or pregnancy-induced hypertension [125]. This study [125] provides reassurance about the cardiovascular safety of utilising kisspeptin to develop treatments for reproductive (and possibly other) disorders.

KISSPEPTIN AND METABOLISM

Conflicting reports about the effects of kisspeptin on metabolism have been reported. In male mice, glucagon increases and insulin decreases hepatic kisspeptin expression [126]. In vitro studies using rodent and human pancreatic cells have shown that at nanmolar concentrations kisspeptin decreases glucose stimulated insulin secretion (GSIS), whilst at higher concentrations it increases GSIS (possibly via a non-K1SSR dependent mechanism) [126,127]. Furthermore, intraperitoneal administration of kisspeptin-10 or kisspeptin-54 to male mice results in impaired glucose tolerance due to reduced GSIS [126]. Administration of an intravenous bolus of kisspeptin-10 to male monkeys does not change basal insulin levels in the fed or fasted states but it results in enhanced GSIS [128].

Ovariectomised female knockout mice that lack the kisspeptin receptor eat less food, have reduced energy expenditure, gain more weight and have impaired glucose homeostasis when compared to ovariectomised wild type mice [129]. However, male kisspeptin receptor knockout mice have similar body weight and glucose tolerance to their wild type littermates [129]. Kisspeptin activates anorectic pro-opiomelanocortin (POMC) and inhibits orexigenic neuropeptide Y (NPY) neurones in hypothalamic tissue from mice [130], whilst conversely in sheep central administration of kisspeptin reduces POMC and increases NPY expression in the hypothalamus [131]. Therefore, differences in sex and species studied, as well as differences in in vitro versus in vivo studies may account for the lack of clarity surrounding kisspeptin's role in metabolism, and more studies (particularly human studies) are required.

THERAPEUTIC POTENTIAL OF KISSPEPTIN

In vitro fertilisation

Following on from the studies that demonstrated that peripheral kisspeptin administration stimulates the pulsatile secretion of reproductive hormones, 2 studies have reported successful use of kisspeptin-54 to trigger egg maturation in women undergoing in vitro fertilisation (IVF) treatment for subfertility. In the first study, the absolute number of mature eggs and oocyte yield appeared to increase in a dose-dependent manner, fertilisation and embryo transfer occurred in 92% of the 53 patients, biochemical pregnancy occurred in 40%, and 10 women had live births (8 singletons and 2 sets of twins) [132]. Adverse events included two ectopic pregnancies, one heterotopic pregnancy and two miscarriages [132]. The second study investigated kisspeptin as a trigger for egg maturation in IVF in women at high (approximately 33%) risk of ovarian hyperstimulation syndrome (OHSS) [a potentially life-threatening condition caused by the long duration of action of hCG, the hormone that is routinely used to trigger egg maturation in IVF] [133]. In this study increasing the dose of kisspeptin did not change the biochemical pregnancy rate (63%), clinical pregnancy rate (53%) and live birth rate per embryo transfer (45%). Adverse events included 4 cases of mild OHSS (no moderate or life-threatening OHSS occurred), 2 ectopic pregnancies, 3 miscarriages and 1 stillbirth at 25 weeks' gestation [133]. Further studies directly comparing the efficacy and safety of kisspeptin-54 and hCG are required to establish how best kisspeptin can be used in IVF.

IHH due to *TAC3/TACR3* mutations

Neurokinin B (NKB) and kisspeptin are co-localised in KNDy neurones [90]. The role of NKB in human reproduction has not been fully characterised but people with inactivating mutations in the genes for NKB (*TAC3*) or its receptor (*TACR3*) exhibit hypogonadotrophic hypogonadism and do not go through puberty. Intravenous kisspeptin-10 restores LH pulsatility and increases FSH pulse frequency in people with these mutations [134]. Therefore, kisspeptin may potentially be used to treat these patients.

Hyperprolactinaemia

In light of the fact that kisspeptin has been shown to restore gonadotrophin secretion in hyperprolactinaemic rodents, kisspeptin may prove to be a useful alternative in treating the hypogonadotrophic hypogonadism caused by hyperprolactinaemia particularly in patients who are intolerant of or are not suitable for dopamine agonist therapy. However, human studies are required to clearly establish if kisspeptin can be used safely and effaciously in hyperprolactinaemic conditions.

Functional hypothalamic amenorrhea

The studies described above in which kisspeptin-54 was used to restore LH pulsatility in women with FHA indicate that kisspeptin may prove to be a promising treatment for this common reproductive disorder. Longer term studies will be necessary to determine if the restoration of LH pulsatility produces regular cycles and restores fertility in this patient group.

Long-term suppression of sex hormones

As described above, desensitisation to the gonadotrophin-stimulating effects of kisspeptin occurs when high kisspeptin doses are used acutely or chronically, and reduced kisspeptin receptor activation results in reduced gonadotrophin and sex hormone release. In Phase II studies, two different kisspeptin receptor analogues have been shown to be well tolerated and suppress testosterone concentrations to below 50 ng/dL in healthy men and men with prostate cancer after 7 days of either a continuous infusion, daily subcutaneous injections or after administration of a 1-month depot formulation [135,136]. Phase III studies will be required before these treatments can be used as licensed therapies.

Cancer treatment

Due to the inverse relationship between *KISS1* expression and metastatic potential, metastasis and clinical outcome observed in some cancers, kisspeptin may prove to be a useful marker for cancers that are less likely to metastasise or be used as a risk stratification tool. Furthermore, kisspeptin levels are elevated in malignant gestational trophoblastic disease and fall to non-pregnant female levels following successful chemotherapy treatment [137], so kisspeptin might represent a novel tumour marker in patients with this disease. Following on from a report that topical imiquimod (a drug that has many actions including increasing *KISS1* expression) produced a 90% regression of skin metastasis in malignant melanoma [138], treatments that upregulate *KISS1* expression may be explored in an attempt to improve outcomes in cancer treatment.

CONCLUSION

Kisspeptin is a relatively recently-discovered hormone, with emerging roles in reproductive, cardiovascular and metabolic systems, as well as in oncology. Ongoing and future research will shed more light on the functions of kisspeptin within these important biological systems and may result in the development of novel therapeutic agents to treat reproductive and malignant disorders.

Key points for clinical practice

- Kisspeptin plays a crucial role in the onset and progression of puberty as well as the maintenance of normal reproductive function.
- Kisspeptin-based therapies have the potential to be used in IVF (both in women who are at low/medium and high risk of OHSS), and in the treatment of reproductive disorders such as FHA and some genetic causes of infertility.
- Kisspeptin analogues (which reduce gonadotrophin and sex hormone levels) are being developed for use in situations where low sex hormone levels are desired such as in hormone sensitive cancer treatment.
- Knowledge about the role of kisspeptin in cardiovascular and metabolic systems is increasing, and this information will prove vital if kisspeptin-based therapies are to be used safely in clinical practice.
- Further research is required before the observed antimetastatic effect of kisspeptin can be harnessed and used as part of the arsenal of treatment for malignancies.

REFERENCES

1. Lee JH, Miele ME, Hicks DJ, et al. KiSS-1, a novel human malignant melanoma metastasis-suppressor gene. J Natl Cancer Inst 1996; 88:1731–1737.
2. Kotani M, Detheux M, Vandenbogaerde A, et al. The metastasis suppressor gene KiSS-1 encodes kisspeptins, the natural ligands of the orphan G protein-coupled receptor GPR54. J Biol Chem 2001; 276:34631–3466.

3. Ohtaki T, Shintani Y, Honda S, et al. Metastasis suppressor gene KiSS-1 encodes peptide ligand of a G-protein-coupled receptor. Nature 2001; 411:613–617.

4. Rometo AM, Krajewski SJ, Voytko ML, Rance NE. Hypertrophy and increased kisspeptin gene expression in the hypothalamic infundibular nucleus of postmenopausal women and ovariectomized monkeys. J Clin Endocrinol Metab 2007; 92:2744–2750.

5. Hrabovszky E, Ciofi P, Vida B, et al. The kisspeptin system of the human hypothalamus: sexual dimorphism and relationship with gonadotropin-releasing hormone and neurokinin B neurons. Eur J Neurosci 2010; 31:1984–1998.

6. Muir AI, Chamberlain L, Elshourbagy NA, et al. AXOR12, a novel human G protein-coupled receptor, activated by the peptide KiSS-1. J Biol Chem 2001; 276:28969–28975.

7. Gaytan F, Gaytán M, Castellano JM, et al. KiSS-1 in the mammalian ovary: distribution of kisspeptin in human and marmoset and alterations in KiSS-1 mRNA levels in a rat model of ovulatory dysfunction. Am J Physiol Endocrinol Metab 2009; 296:E520–531.

8. Garcia-Ortega J, Pinto FM, Fernández-Sánchez M, et al. Expression of neurokinin B/NK3 receptor and kisspeptin/KISS1 receptor in human granulosa cells. Hum Reprod 2014; 29:2736–2746.

9. Cejudo Roman A, Pinto FM, Dorta I, et al. Analysis of the expression of neurokinin B, kisspeptin, and their cognate receptors NK3R and KISS1R in the human female genital tract. Fertil Steril 2012; 97:1213–1219.

10. Takahashi K, Shoji I, Shibasaki A, et al. Presence of kisspeptin-like immunoreactivity in human adrenal glands and adrenal tumors. J Mol Neurosci 2010; 41:138–144.

11. Lee DK, Nguyen T, O'Neill GP, et al. Discovery of a receptor related to the galanin receptors. FEBS Lett 1999; 446:103–107.

12. Nakamura Y, Aoki S, Xing Y, Sasano H, Rainey WE. Metastin stimulates aldosterone synthesis in human adrenal cells. Reprod Sci 2007; 14:836–845.

13. Kallo I, Vida B, Deli L, Molnár CS, et al. Co-localisation of kisspeptin with galanin or neurokinin B in afferents to mouse GnRH neurones. J Neuroendocrinol 2012; 24:464–476.

14. Irwig MS, Fraley GS, Smith JT, et al. Kisspeptin activation of gonadotropin releasing hormone neurons and regulation of KiSS-1 mRNA in the male rat. Neuroendocrinology 2004; 80:264–272.

15. Thompson EL, Patterson M, Murphy KG, et al. Central and peripheral administration of kisspeptin-10 stimulates the hypothalamic-pituitary-gonadal axis. J Neuroendocrinol 2004; 16:850–858.

16. Messager S, Chatzidaki EE, Ma D, et al. Kisspeptin directly stimulates gonadotropin-releasing hormone release via G protein-coupled receptor 54. Proc Natl Acad Sci U S A 2005; 102:1761–1766.

17. d'Anglemont de Tassigny X, Fagg LA, Carlton MB, Colledge WH. Kisspeptin can stimulate gonadotropin-releasing hormone (GnRH) release by a direct action at GnRH nerve terminals. Endocrinology 2008; 149:3926–3932.

18. Dhillo WS, Chaudhri OB, Patterson M, et al. Kisspeptin-54 stimulates the hypothalamic-pituitary gonadal axis in human males. J Clin Endocrinol Metab 2005; 90:6609–6615.

19. Smith JT, Rao A, Pereira A, et al. Kisspeptin is present in ovine hypophysial portal blood but does not increase during the preovulatory luteinizing hormone surge: evidence that gonadotropes are not direct targets of kisspeptin in vivo. Endocrinology 2008; 149:1951–1959.

20. Jayasena CN, Comninos AN, Narayanaswamy S, et al. Acute and chronic effects of kisspeptin-54 administration on GH, prolactin and TSH secretion in healthy women. Clin Endocrinol (Oxf) 2014; 81:891–898.

21. Smith JT, Cunningham MJ, Rissman EF, Clifton DK, Steiner RA. Regulation of Kiss1 gene expression in the brain of the female mouse. Endocrinology 2005; 146:3686–3692.

22. Smith JT, Dungan HM, Stoll EA, et al. Differential regulation of KiSS-1 mRNA expression by sex steroids in the brain of the male mouse. Endocrinology 2005; 146:2976–2984.

23. George JT, Anderson RA, Millar RP. Kisspeptin-10 stimulation of gonadotrophin secretion in women is modulated by sex steroid feedback. Hum Reprod 2012; 27:3552–3559.

24. Wintermantel TM, Campbell RE, Porteous R, et al. Definition of estrogen receptor pathway critical for estrogen positive feedback to gonadotropin-releasing hormone neurons and fertility. Neuron 2006; 52:271–280.

25. Hrabovszky E, Shughrue PJ, Merchenthaler I, et al. Detection of estrogen receptor-beta messenger ribonucleic acid and 125I-estrogen binding sites in luteinizing hormone-releasing hormone neurons of the rat brain. Endocrinology 2000; 141:3506–3509.

26. Herbison AE, Pape JR. New evidence for estrogen receptors in gonadotropin-releasing hormone neurons. Front Neuroendocrinol 2001; 22:292–308.

27. Roa J, Vigo E, Castellano JM, et al. Opposite roles of estrogen receptor (ER)-alpha and ERbeta in the modulation of luteinizing hormone responses to kisspeptin in the female rat: implications for the generation of the preovulatory surge. Endocrinology 2008; 149:1627–1637.

28. Redmond JS, Macedo GG, Velez IC, et al. Kisspeptin activates the hypothalamic-adenohypophyseal-gonadal axis in prepubertal ewe lambs. Reproduction 2011; 141:541–548.

29. Nestor CC, Briscoe AM, Davis SM, et al. Evidence of a role for kisspeptin and neurokinin B in puberty of female sheep. Endocrinology 2012; 153:2756–2765.

30. Guerriero KA, Keen KL, Terasawa E. Developmental increase in kisspeptin-54 release in vivo is independent of the pubertal increase in estradiol in female rhesus monkeys (Macaca mulatta). Endocrinology 2012; 153:1887–1897.

31. Navarro VM, Fernández-Fernández R, Castellano JM, et al. Advanced vaginal opening and precocious activation of the reproductive axis by KiSS-1 peptide, the endogenous ligand of GPR54. J Physiol 2004; 561:379–386.

32. Silveira LG, Noel SD, Silveira-Neto AP, et al. Mutations of the KISS1 gene in disorders of puberty. J Clin Endocrinol Metab 2010; 95:2276–2280.

33. Teles MG, Bianco SD, Brito VN, et al. A GPR54-activating mutation in a patient with central precocious puberty. N Engl J Med 2008; 358:709–715.

34. Pita J, Barrios V, Gavela-Pérez T, et al. Circulating kisspeptin levels exhibit sexual dimorphism in adults, are increased in obese prepubertal girls and do not suffer modifications in girls with idiopathic central precocious puberty. Peptides 2011; 32:1781–1786.

35. Jayasena CN, Nijher GM, Narayanaswamy S, et al. Age-dependent elevations in plasma kisspeptin are observed in boys and girls when compared with adults. Ann Clin Biochem 2014; 51:89–96.

36. Topaloglu AK, Tello JA, Kotan LD, et al. Inactivating KISS1 mutation and hypogonadotropic hypogonadism. N Engl J Med 2012; 366:629–635.

37. Seminara SB, Messager S, Chatzidaki E, et al. The GPR54 gene as a regulator of puberty. N Engl J Med 2003; 349:1614–1627.

38. de Roux N, Genin E, Carel JC, et al. Hypogonadotropic hypogonadism due to loss of function of the KiSS1-derived peptide receptor GPR54. Proc Natl Acad Sci 2003; 100:10972–10976.

39. Nimri R, Lebenthal Y, Lazar L, et al. A novel loss-of-function mutation in GPR54/KISS1R leads to hypogonadotropic hypogonadism in a highly consanguineous family. J Clin Endocrinol Metab 2011; 96:E536–545.

40. George JT, Veldhuis JD, Roseweir AK, et al. Kisspeptin-10 is a potent stimulator of LH and increases pulse frequency in men. J Clin Endocrinol Metab 2011; 96:E1228–1236.

41. Jayasena CN, Nijher GM, Comninos AN, et al. The effects of kisspeptin-10 on reproductive hormone release show sexual dimorphism in humans. J Clin Endocrinol Metab 2011; 96:E1963–1972.

42. Chan YM, Butler JP, Pinnell NE, et al. Kisspeptin resets the hypothalamic GnRH clock in men. J Clin Endocrinol Metab 2011; 96:E908–915.

43. George JT, Veldhuis JD, Tena-Sempere M, Millar RP, Anderson RA. Exploring the pathophysiology of hypogonadism in men with type 2 diabetes: kisspeptin-10 stimulates serum testosterone and LH secretion in men with type 2 diabetes and mild biochemical hypogonadism. Clin Endocrinol (Oxf) 2013; 79:100–104.

44. Jayasena CN, Abbara A, Narayanaswamy S, et al. Direct comparison of the effects of intravenous kisspeptin-10, kisspeptin-54 and GnRH on gonadotrophin secretion in healthy men. Hum Reprod 2015; 30:1934–1941.

45. Dhillo WS, Chaudhri OB, Thompson EL, et al. Kisspeptin-54 stimulates gonadotropin release most potently during the preovulatory phase of the menstrual cycle in women. J Clin Endocrinol Metab 2007; 92:3958–3966.

46. Jayasena CN, Comninos AN, Nijher GM, et al. Twice-daily subcutaneous injection of kisspeptin-54 does not abolish menstrual cyclicity in healthy female volunteers. J Clin Endocrinol Metab 2013; 98:4464–4474.

47. Narayanaswamy S, Jayasena CN, Ng N, et al. Subcutaneous infusion of kisspeptin-54 stimulates gonadotrophin release in women and the response correlates with basal oestradiol levels. Clin Endocrinol (Oxf), 2015.

48. Jayasena CN, Comninos AN, Narayanaswamy S, et al. The identification of elevated urinary kisspeptin-immunoreactivity during pregnancy. Ann Clin Biochem 2015; 52:395–398.

49. Horikoshi Y, Matsumoto H, Takatsu Y, et al. Dramatic elevation of plasma metastin concentrations in human pregnancy: metastin as a novel placenta-derived hormone in humans. J Clin Endocrinol Metab 2003; 88:914–919.

50. Jayasena CN, Abbara A, Izzi-Engbeaya C, et al. Reduced levels of plasma kisspeptin during the antenatal booking visit are associated with increased risk of miscarriage. J Clin Endocrinol Metab 2014; 99:E2652–2660.

51. Logie JJ, Denison FC, Riley SC, et al. Evaluation of kisspeptin levels in obese pregnancy as a biomarker for pre-eclampsia. Clin Endocrinol (Oxf), 2012; 76:887–893.

52. Cetkovic A, Miljic D, Ljubić A, et al. Plasma kisspeptin levels in pregnancies with diabetes and hypertensive disease as a potential marker of placental dysfunction and adverse perinatal outcome. Endocr Res 2012; 37:78–88.

53. Madazli R, Bulut B, Tuten A, et al. First-trimester maternal serum metastin, placental growth factor and chitotriosidase levels in pre-eclampsia. Eur J Obstet Gynecol Reprod Biol 2012; 164:146–149.

54. Kavvasoglu S, Ozkan ZS, Kumbak B, Sımsek M, Ilhan N. Association of kisspeptin-10 levels with abortus imminens: a preliminary study. Arch Gynecol Obstet 2012; 285:649–653.

55. Adali E, Kurdoglu Z, Kurdoglu M, et al. Metastin levels in pregnancies complicated by pre-eclampsia and their relation with disease severity. J Matern Fetal Neonatal Med 2012; 25:2671–2675.

56. Janneau JL, Maldonado-Estrada J, Tachdjian G, et al. Transcriptional expression of genes involved in cell invasion and migration by normal and tumoral trophoblast cells. J Clin Endocrinol Metab 2002; 87:5336–5339.

57. Bilban M, Ghaffari-Tabrizi N, Hintermann E, et al. Kisspeptin-10, a KiSS-1/metastin-derived decapeptide, is a physiological invasion inhibitor of primary human trophoblasts. J Cell Sci 2004; 117:1319–1328.

58. Taylor J, Pampillo M, Bhattacharya M, Babwah AV. Kisspeptin/KISS1R signaling potentiates extravillous trophoblast adhesion to type-I collagen in a PKC- and ERK1/2-dependent manner. Mol Reprod Dev 2014; 81:42–54.

59. Ramaesh T, Logie JJ, Roseweir AK, et al. Kisspeptin-10 inhibits angiogenesis in human placental vessels ex vivo and endothelial cells in vitro. Endocrinology 2010; 151:5927–5934.

60. Park DW, Lee SK, Hong SR, et al. Expression of Kisspeptin and its receptor GPR54 in the first trimester trophoblast of women with recurrent pregnancy loss. Am J Reprod Immunol 2012; 67:132–139.

61. Wu S, Tian J1, Liu L, et al. Expression of kisspeptin/GPR54 and PIBF/PR in the first trimester trophoblast and decidua of women with recurrent spontaneous abortion. Pathol Res Pract 2014; 210:47–54.

62. Cartwright JE, Williams PJ. Altered placental expression of kisspeptin and its receptor in pre-eclampsia. J Endocrinol 2012; 214:79–85.

63. Zhang H, Long Q, Ling L, et al. Elevated expression of KiSS-1 in placenta of preeclampsia and its effect on trophoblast. Reprod Biol 2011; 11:99–115.

64. Vazquez-Alaniz F, Galaviz-Hernandez C, Marchat LA, et al. Comparative expression profiles for KiSS-1 and REN genes in preeclamptic and healthy placental tissues. Eur J Obstet Gynecol Reprod Biol 2011; 159:67–71.

65. Kokay IC, Petersen SL, Grattan DR. Identification of prolactin-sensitive GABA and kisspeptin neurons in regions of the rat hypothalamus involved in the control of fertility. Endocrinology 2011; 152:526–535.

66. Brown RS, Herbison AE, Grattan DR. Prolactin regulation of kisspeptin neurones in the mouse brain and its role in the lactation-induced suppression of kisspeptin expression. J Neuroendocrinol, 2014; 26:898–908.

67. Araujo-Lopes R, Crampton JR, Aquino NS, et al. Prolactin regulates kisspeptin neurons in the arcuate nucleus to suppress LH secretion in female rats. Endocrinology 2014; 155:1010–1020.

68. Sonigo C, Bouilly J, Carré N, et al. Hyperprolactinemia-induced ovarian acyclicity is reversed by kisspeptin administration. J Clin Invest 2012; 122:3791–3795.

69. Ribeiro AB, Leite CM, Kalil B, et al. Kisspeptin regulates tuberoinfundibular dopaminergic neurones and prolactin secretion in an oestradiol-dependent manner in male and female rats. J Neuroendocrinol 2015; 27:88–99.

70. Szawka RE, Ribeiro AB, Leite CM, et al. Kisspeptin regulates prolactin release through hypothalamic dopaminergic neurons. Endocrinology 2010; 151:3247–3257.

71. Ramaswamy S, Gibbs RB, Plant TM. Studies of the localisation of kisspeptin within the pituitary of the rhesus monkey (Macaca mulatta) and the effect of kisspeptin on the release of non-gonadotropic pituitary hormones. J Neuroendocrinol 2009; 21:795–804.

72. Liu JH, Patel B, Collins G. Central Causes of Amenorrhea. Endotext, 2016.

73. Jayasena CN, Nijher GM, Chaudhri OB, et al. Subcutaneous injection of kisspeptin-54 acutely stimulates gonadotropin secretion in women with hypothalamic amenorrhea, but chronic administration causes tachyphylaxis. J Clin Endocrinol Metab 2009; 94:4315–4323.

74. Jayasena CN, Abbara A, Veldhuis JD, et al. Increasing LH pulsatility in women with hypothalamic amenorrhoea using intravenous infusion of Kisspeptin-54. J Clin Endocrinol Metab 2014; 99:E953–961.

75. Jayasena CN, Nijher GM, Abbara A, et al. Twice-weekly administration of kisspeptin-54 for 8 weeks stimulates release of reproductive hormones in women with hypothalamic amenorrhea. Clin Pharmacol Ther 2010; 88:840–847.

76. Zhang Y, Proenca R, Maffei M, et al. Positional cloning of the mouse obese gene and its human homologue. Nature 1994; 372:425–432.

77. Frederich RC, Löllmann B, Hamann A, et al. Expression of ob mRNA and its encoded protein in rodents. Impact of nutrition and obesity. J Clin Invest 1995; 96:1658–1663.

78. Maffei M, Halaas J, Ravussin E, et al. Leptin levels in human and rodent: measurement of plasma leptin and ob RNA in obese and weight-reduced subjects. Nat Med 1995; 1:1155–1161.

79. Sinha MK, Opentanova I, Ohannesian JP, et al. Evidence of free and bound leptin in human circulation. Studies in lean and obese subjects and during short-term fasting. J Clin Invest 1996; 98:1277–1282.

80. Smith JT, Acohido BV, Clifton DK, Steiner RA. KiSS-1 neurones are direct targets for leptin in the ob/ob mouse. J Neuroendocrinol 2006; 18:298–303.

81. Quennell JH, Mulligan AC, Tups A, et al. Leptin indirectly regulates gonadotropin-releasing hormone neuronal function. Endocrinology 2009; 150:2805–2812.

82. Bray GA, York DA. Genetically transmitted obesity in rodents. Physiol Rev 1971; 51:598–646.

83. Chehab FF, Lim ME, Lu R. Correction of the sterility defect in homozygous obese female mice by treatment with the human recombinant leptin. Nat Genet 1996; 12:318–320.

84. Strobel A, Issad T, Camoin L, Ozata M, Strosberg AD. A leptin missense mutation associated with hypogonadism and morbid obesity. Nat Genet 1998; 18:213–215.

85. Farooqi IS, Matarese G, Lord GM, et al. Beneficial effects of leptin on obesity, T cell hyporesponsiveness, and neuroendocrine/metabolic dysfunction of human congenital leptin deficiency. J Clin Invest 2002; 110:1093–1103.

86. Laughlin GA, Yen SS. Hypoleptinemia in women athletes: absence of a diurnal rhythm with amenorrhea. J Clin Endocrinol Metab 1997; 82:318–321.

87. Welt CK, Chan JL, Bullen J, et al. Recombinant human leptin in women with hypothalamic amenorrhea. N Engl J Med 2004; 351:987–997.

88. Kanasaki H, Purwana IN, Oride A, et al. Circulating kisspeptin and pituitary adenylate cyclase-activating polypeptide (PACAP) do not correlate with gonadotropin serum levels. Gynecol Endocrinol 2013; 29:583–587.

89. Peng J, Xu H, Yang B, et al. Plasma levels of kisspeptins in postmenopausal Chinese women do not show substantial elevation. Peptides 2010; 31:2255–2258.

90. Goodman RL, Lehman MN, Smith JT, et al. Kisspeptin neurons in the arcuate nucleus of the ewe express both dynorphin A and neurokinin B. Endocrinology 2007; 148:5752–5760.

91. Mittelman-Smith MA, Williams H, Krajewski-Hall SJ, et al. Arcuate kisspeptin/neurokinin B/dynorphin (KNDy) neurons mediate the estrogen suppression of gonadotropin secretion and body weight. Endocrinology 2012; 153:2800–2812.

92. Rance NE, Dacks PA, Mittelman-Smith MA, et al. Modulation of body temperature and LH secretion by hypothalamic KNDy (kisspeptin, neurokinin B and dynorphin) neurons: a novel hypothesis on the mechanism of hot flushes. Front Neuroendocrinol 2013; 34:211–227.

93. Lee JH, Welch DR. Suppression of metastasis in human breast carcinoma MDA-MB-435 cells after transfection with the metastasis suppressor gene, KiSS-1. Cancer Res 1997; 57:2384–2387.

94. Martins CM, Fernandes BF, Antecka E, et al. Expression of the metastasis suppressor gene KISS1 in uveal melanoma. Eye (Lond) 2008; 22:707–711.

95. Dhar DK, Naora H, Kubota H, et al. Downregulation of KiSS-1 expression is responsible for tumor invasion and worse prognosis in gastric carcinoma. Int J Cancer 2004; 111:868–872.

96. Ikeguchi M, Yamaguchi K, Kaibara N. Clinical significance of the loss of KiSS-1 and orphan G-protein-coupled receptor (hOT7T175) gene expression in esophageal squamous cell carcinoma. Clin Cancer Res 2004; 10:1379–1383.

97. Wang W, Yang ZL, Liu JQ, et al. Overexpression of MTA1 and loss of KAI-1 and KiSS-1 expressions are associated with invasion, metastasis, and poor-prognosis of gallbladder adenocarcinoma. Tumori 2014; 100:667–674.

98. Sanchez-Carbayo M, Capodieci P, Cordon-Cardo C. Tumor suppressor role of KiSS-1 in bladder cancer: loss of KiSS-1 expression is associated with bladder cancer progression and clinical outcome. Am J Pathol 2003; 162:609–617.

99. Stark AM, Tongers K, Maass N, Mehdorn HM, Held-Feindt J. Reduced metastasis-suppressor gene mRNA-expression in breast cancer brain metastases. J Cancer Res Clin Oncol 2005; 131:191–198.

100. Nagai K, Doi R, Katagiri F, et al. Prognostic value of metastin expression in human pancreatic cancer. J Exp Clin Cancer Res 2009; 28:9.

101. Zheng S, Chang Y, Hodges KB, et al. Expression of KISS1 and MMP-9 in non-small cell lung cancer and their relations to metastasis and survival. Anticancer Res 2010; 30:713–718.
102. Chen Y, Yusenko MV, Kovacs G. Lack of KISS1R expression is associated with rapid progression of conventional renal cell carcinomas. J Pathol 2011; 223:46–53.
103. Okugawa Y, Inoue Y, Tanaka K. et al. Loss of the metastasis suppressor gene KiSS1 is associated with lymph node metastasis and poor prognosis in human colorectal cancer. Oncol Rep 2013; 30:1449–1454.
104. Yuan TZ, Zhang HH, Tang QF, et al. Prognostic value of kisspeptin expression in nasopharyngeal carcinoma. Laryngoscope 2014; 124:E167–174.
105. Hata K, Dhar DK, Watanabe Y, Nakai H, Hoshiai H. Expression of metastin and a G-protein-coupled receptor (AXOR12) in epithelial ovarian cancer. Eur J Cancer 2007; 43:1452–1459.
106. Prentice LM, Klausen C, Kalloger S, et al. Kisspeptin and GPR54 immunoreactivity in a cohort of 518 patients defines favourable prognosis and clear cell subtype in ovarian carcinoma. BMC Med 2007; 5:33.
107. Ikeguchi M, Hirooka Y, Kaibara N. Quantitative reverse transcriptase polymerase chain reaction analysis for KiSS-1 and orphan G-protein-coupled receptor (hOT7T175) gene expression in hepatocellular carcinoma. J Cancer Res Clin Oncol 2003; 129:531–535.
108. Schmid K, Wang X, Haitel A, et al. KiSS-1 overexpression as an independent prognostic marker in hepatocellular carcinoma: an immunohistochemical study. Virchows Arch 2007; 450:143–149.
109. Kostakis ID, Agrogiannis G, Vaiopoulos AG, et al. KISS1 expression in colorectal cancer. APMIS 2013; 121:1004–1010.
110. Kostakis ID, Agrogiannis G, Vaiopoulos AG, et al. A clinicopathological analysis of KISS1 and KISS1R expression in colorectal cancer. APMIS 2015; 123:629–637.
111. Martin TA, Watkins G, Jiang WG. KiSS-1 expression in human breast cancer. Clin Exp Metastasis 2005; 22:503–511.
112. Marot D, Bieche I, Aumas C, et al. High tumoral levels of Kiss1 and G-protein-coupled receptor 54 expression are correlated with poor prognosis of estrogen receptor-positive breast tumors. Endocr Relat Cancer 2007; 14:691–702.
113. Masui T, Doi R, Mori T, et al. Metastin and its variant forms suppress migration of pancreatic cancer cells. Biochem Biophys Res Commun 2004; 315:85–92.
114. Jiang Y, Berk M, Singh LS, et al. KiSS1 suppresses metastasis in human ovarian cancer via inhibition of protein kinase C alpha. Clin Exp Metastasis 2005; 22:369–376.
115. Shoji S, Tang XY, Umemura S, et al. Metastin inhibits migration and invasion of renal cell carcinoma with overexpression of metastin receptor. Eur Urol 2009; 55:441–449.
116. Li N, Wang HX, Zhang J, Ye YP, He GY. KISS-1 inhibits the proliferation and invasion of gastric carcinoma cells. World J Gastroenterol 2012; 18:1827–1833.
117. Wang H, Jones J, Turner T, et al. Clinical and biological significance of KISS1 expression in prostate cancer. Am J Pathol 2012; 180:1170–1178.
118. Zhang Y, Tang YJ, Li ZH, et al. KiSS1 inhibits growth and invasion of osteosarcoma cells through inhibition of the MAPK pathway. Eur J Histochem 2013; 57:e30.
119. Becker JA, Mirjolet JF, Bernard J, et al. Activation of GPR54 promotes cell cycle arrest and apoptosis of human tumor cells through a specific transcriptional program not shared by other Gq-coupled receptors. Biochem Biophys Res Commun 2005; 326:677–686.
120. Cho SG, Yi Z, Pang X, et al. Kisspeptin-10, a KISS1-derived decapeptide, inhibits tumor angiogenesis by suppressing Sp1-mediated VEGF expression and FAK/Rho GTPase activation. Cancer Res 2009; 69:7062–7070.
121. Ji K, Ye L, Ruge F, et al. Implication of metastasis suppressor gene, Kiss-1 and its receptor Kiss-1R in colorectal cancer. BMC Cancer 2014; 14:723.
122. Schmidt E, Haase M, Ziegler E, Emons G, Gründker C. Kisspeptin-10 inhibits stromal-derived factor 1-induced invasion of human endometrial cancer cells. Int J Gynecol Cancer 2014; 24:210–217.
123. Maguire JJ, Kirby HR, Mead EJ, et al. Inotropic action of the puberty hormone kisspeptin in rat, mouse and human: cardiovascular distribution and characteristics of the kisspeptin receptor. PLoS One 2011; 6:e27601.
124. Mead EJ, Maguire JJ, Kuc RE, Davenport AP. Kisspeptins are novel potent vasoconstrictors in humans, with a discrete localization of their receptor, G protein-coupled receptor 54, to atherosclerosis-prone vessels. Endocrinology 2007; 148:140–147.
125. Nijher GM, Chaudhri OB, Ramachandran R, et al. The effects of kisspeptin-54 on blood pressure in humans and plasma kisspeptin concentrations in hypertensive diseases of pregnancy. Br J Clin Pharmacol 2010; 70:674–681.

126. Song WJ, Mondal P, Wolfe A et al. Glucagon regulates hepatic kisspeptin to impair insulin secretion. Cell Metab 2014; 19:667–681.

127. Bowe JE, Foot VL, Amiel SA, et al. GPR54 peptide agonists stimulate insulin secretion from murine, porcine and human islets. Islets 2012; 4:20–23.

128. Wahab F, Riaz T, Shahab M. Study on the effect of peripheral kisspeptin administration on basal and glucose-induced insulin secretion under fed and fasting conditions in the adult male rhesus monkey (Macaca mulatta). Horm Metab Res 2011; 43:37–42.

129. Tolson KP, Garcia C, Yen S, et al. Impaired kisspeptin signaling decreases metabolism and promotes glucose intolerance and obesity. J Clin Invest 2014; 124:3075–3079.

130. Fu LY, van den Pol AN. Kisspeptin directly excites anorexigenic proopiomelanocortin neurons but inhibits orexigenic neuropeptide Y cells by an indirect synaptic mechanism. J Neurosci 2010; 30:10205–10219.

131. Backholer K, Smith JT, Rao A, et al. Kisspeptin cells in the ewe brain respond to leptin and communicate with neuropeptide Y and proopiomelanocortin cells. Endocrinology, 2010; 151:2233–2243.

132. Jayasena CN, Abbara A, Comninos AN, et al. Kisspeptin-54 triggers egg maturation in women undergoing in vitro fertilization. J Clin Invest 2014; 124:3667–3677.

133. Abbara A, Jayasena CN1, Christopoulos G, et al. Efficacy of Kisspeptin-54 to Trigger Oocyte Maturation in Women at High Risk of Ovarian Hyperstimulation Syndrome (OHSS) During In Vitro Fertilization (IVF) Therapy. J Clin Endocrinol Metab 2015; 100:3322–3331.

134. Young J, George JT, Tello JA, et al. Kisspeptin restores pulsatile LH secretion in patients with neurokinin B signaling deficiencies: physiological, pathophysiological and therapeutic implications. Neuroendocrinology 2013; 97:193–202.

135. MacLean DB, Matsui H, Suri A, Neuwirth R, Colombel M. Sustained exposure to the investigational Kisspeptin analog, TAK-448, down-regulates testosterone into the castration range in healthy males and in patients with prostate cancer: results from two phase 1 studies. J Clin Endocrinol Metab 2014; 99:E1445–1453.

136. Scott G, Ahmad I, Howard K, et al. Double-blind, randomized, placebo-controlled study of safety, tolerability, pharmacokinetics and pharmacodynamics of TAK-683, an investigational metastin analogue in healthy men. Br J Clin Pharmacol 2013; 75:381–91.

137. Dhillo WS, Savage P, Murphy KG, et al. Plasma kisspeptin is raised in patients with gestational trophoblastic neoplasia and falls during treatment. Am J Physiol Endocrinol Metab 2006; 291:E878–884.

138. Hesling C, D'Incan M, Mansard S, et al. In vivo and in situ modulation of the expression of genes involved in metastasis and angiogenesis in a patient treated with topical imiquimod for melanoma skin metastases. Br J Dermatol 2004; 150:761–767.

The second agent licensed for the treatment of obesity in the UK was liraglutide, a once-daily, long-acting glucagon-like peptide (GLP-1) analogue. This was approved for the treatment of obesity in March 2015, although to date it has not been marketed. GLP-1 is released by the L-cells of the small intestine and colon and the alpha cells of the Islets of Langerhans in response to food intake [23,24]. GLP-1 analogues were originally used in the treatment of type 2 diabetes because GLP-1 is an endogenous incretin, which acts to augment glucose dependent insulin secretion and suppress glucagon release [25]. The rationale for their use in the treatment of obesity is two-fold. Firstly, GLP-1 has an anorectic effect in humans [26] and when exogenously administered, this effect is seen to be preserved in obese subjects [27]. Various mechanisms have been proposed for this pro-satiety effect, including effects on the afferent vagus nerve [28] and binding to the GLP-1 receptor in central nervous system areas known to be important in the modulation of food intake such as the arcuate nucleus, the paraventricular nucleus and the supraoptic nucleus of the hypothalamus (29–31) and the nucleus of the solitary tract (NTS) of the brain stem [32]. Secondly, GLP-1 has been shown to reduce the rate of gastric emptying [33], an effect which might also contribute to the reduction in food intake. Both the anorectic effect of GLP-1 and the slowing of gastric emptying are abolished by vagal afferent denervation [34,35]. Although a proportion of patients experience nausea during liraglutide treatment, this tends to abate with on-going use (Astrup et al. 2009) [36] and patients who did not report nausea also lose weight [37]. GLP-1 agonists are usually best tolerated if a dose titration approach is employed. In the recently published SCALE trial [38], high-dose liraglutide (3 mg once a day) administered to non-diabetic overweight (BMI $\geq$ 27 kg/m^2 with co-morbidity) or obese (BMI > 30 kg/m^2) subjects for 56 weeks found a 5.6-kg placebo subtracted weight loss over the course of the study, however most of the obese patients remained obese and following discontinuation of liraglutide, subjects re-gained 2.9 kg in 12 weeks. This implies that liraglutide therapy, like the treatment for many chronic metabolic diseases such as diabetes and dyslipidaemia, may have to continue indefinitely in order to continue to reap the therapeutic rewards.

Other GLP-1 agonists are currently available for the treatment of type 2 diabetes, e.g. exenatide, dulaglitude and semaglutide. Given the potential rewards of the obesity drug market, it is certainly conceivable that in the future some of these agents will be trialled and licenses sought for use as anti-obesity therapies.

Lastly, a combination of naltrexone and bupropion has recently gained approval for use in the treatment of obesity from both the US Food and Drug Administration (FDA) and the European Medicines Agency (EMA). As a monotherapy, both are indicated for other uses and their weight loss properties were fortuitously discovered. Bupropion is a dopamine/ norepinephrine re-uptake inhibitor used in the treatment of depression and smoking cessation which may increase the firing of the anorectic pro-opiomelanocortin (POMC) neurons of the hypothalamus [39], whilst naltrexone is an opioid receptor antagonist used in the treatment of addiction. Neither has been found to be an efficacious monotherapy for weight loss [40] but when combined four large clinical trials have reported a placebo subtracted mean weight loss of 4.6% or 4.9 kg at 1 year [41-44]. The drop-out rate in these trials was high, at 42–50% of patients, with 24% of the subjects withdrawing because of an adverse event, nausea being the most common. Approval for the drug was conditional on further post-marketing studies to establish the agent's safety, however, the post-market LIGHT study of nearly 9,000 overweight and obese patients was halted in March 2015 and was terminated 2 months later after a partial release of data that occurred without the sanction of the trial lead investigators. A new cardiovascular outcomes trial is anticipated to start later this year, with a projected completion date of 2022.

DRUGS USED TO TREAT OBESITY IN THE USA

Five drugs are currently available in the USA for the treatment of obesity: orlistat, liraglutide, bupropion/naltrexone, lorcaserin and phentermine/topiramate. Orlistat, liraglutide and bupropion/naltrexone have been discussed above; other are discussed here.

Lorcaserin is a 5-HT$_{2C}$ receptor agonist which acts centrally to promote satiety. It was given approval by the FDA in 2012. A meta-analysis of 5 RCTs has shown a mean weight loss of 3.2 kg at 1 year [44], however weight gain in year 2 has been reported [45]. The selectivity at 5HT$_{2C}$ was thought to confer the advantage of not inducing the valvular disease seen with fenfluramine. In 2013, lorcaserin's application for marketing authorisation in Europe was withdrawn [46] following concerns from the EMA about the potential risk of tumours, valvulopathy and psychiatric disorders. By contrast, the FDA's interpretation of the data was that the female rats that developed mammary adenocarcinomas in trials of lorcaserin had a plasma exposure of 87 times the daily human clinical dose, that the increase of mammary fibroadenoma at all doses was of uncertain clinical significance and that safety concerns should be assessed by post-marketing studies [47]. It is not clear whether a re-application to the EMA for European approval is imminent.

The FDA's approval of lorcaserin was followed by its approval of low-dose combined phentermine and topiramate. Topiramate is an anticonvulsant which was noticed to have an appetite suppressive effect. The pro-satiety effects of topiramate are not completely understood and several mechanisms have been postulated including changes in the neurotransmission of the centrally acting orexigen neuropeptide Y (NPY) and peripheral insulin sensitisation [48]. Two large clinical trials showed a 10% weight loss from baseline in the phentermine/topiramate group compared with an under 2% loss in the placebo group [49,50] and this was largely maintained at 2 years [51].

Nevertheless, phentermine/topiramate failed to gain approval from the EMA [52] because of concerns over its cardiovascular safety based on a reported increase in pulse rate, a 4.2% incidence of arrhythmia (versus 1.8% in the placebo group) and six adverse cardiovascular outcomes in the 743 patients taking phentermine/topiramate compared with none in 227 placebo patients. Moreover use of phentermine/topiramate was associated with metabolic acidosis, nephrolithiasis and cognitive defects.

Discrepancies between the FDA and EMA positions on lorcaserin and phentermine/topiramate have been the subject of comment in the medical press [53] with one group of authors stating that both lorcaserin and phentermine/topiramate represent 'slim pickings for the treatment of obesity' concluding that 'until there is more convincing evidence about the cardiovascular safety of these drugs, physicians and patients should approach them with caution' [54], claims that were subsequently refuted by representatives from two obesity organisations [55,56].

THE FUTURE

The quest to develop safe and efficacious treatments for obesity continues. Gastric bypass surgery was initially developed in order to mechanically alter food intake and reduce absorption. It is now accepted that the mechanism of satiety produced by bypass results from an alteration in the secretion of multiple gut hormones. Single hormone therapies such as a lone GLP-1 agonist do not produce weight loss that is comparable to that seen following surgery and the high doses that are required of multiple single agents frequently produce side effects.

From these observations the concept of 'medical bypass' was born, the idea that it may be possible to re-create the gut hormone effects of bariatric surgery without the need for the operation itself. This has led to the development of single-molecule hybrids of either two or three gut hormone receptor agonists in order to augment the effects of singly administered gut hormone analogues and to mimic the synergistic effects of multiple gut hormones working in concert after surgery. Both dual and triple agonist combinations are now in early pre-clinical trials.

Previous work has looked at combining a glucagon receptor agonist (GCGR) which has a pro-energy expenditure effect with a GLP-1 receptor (GLP-1R) agonist that induces satiety and because of its incretin effect, should theoretically offset any potential risk of hyperglycaemia triggered by GCGR. In this work, a set of GCGR/GLP-1R co-agonists were developed and two were chosen for administration to diet-induced obese (DIO) mice once a week for 1 month. These co-agonists produced weight loss of between 20.1% and 28.1% (depending on the co-agonist), reduced food intake and increased energy expenditure all without inducing hyperglycaemia [57]. Subsequently a dual agonist combining agonist action at GLP-1R and the incretin glucose-dependent insulinotropic polypeptide receptor (GIPR) has produced weight loss in rodents [58]. More recently, a tri-agonist at three gut hormone receptors: GLP-1R, GCGR and GIPR has been developed [59]. Administration of the tri-agonist to DIO mice resulted in a 26.6% weight loss over 20 days, accompanied by a dose-dependent reduction in food intake and improvement in glycaemic control, outcomes which were significantly better than those following administration of any of the mono-agonists alone [59]. Whether dual or tri-agonist monomeric peptides survive clinical trials, have an acceptable side effect profile and produce the same efficacy in humans as in mice without rebound, tachyphylaxis or wearing off remains to be determined. In addition, it remains to be seen whether the idea of a 'medical bypass' drug that is an injection and which may be a life-long treatment is acceptable to patients.

A second approach follows on from the cloning of the *ob* gene in 1994 and the demonstration that it encoded an adipocyte-derived hormone, leptin [60], a finding which heralded a new era in obesity research. Leptin is synthesised and secreted by adipocytes signalling information about energy stores and nutritional status [60,61]. Serum leptin levels are proportional to fat mass and fall in both humans and mice after weight loss [62]. The administration of leptin results in a reduction in food intake and body weight [61] through actions on leptin receptors which are found in brain areas known to modulate food intake. In humans a highly significant correlation between body fat content and plasma leptin concentration has been observed and obese humans generally have high leptin levels [63,64]. These data suggest that in most cases, human obesity is likely to be associated with insensitivity to leptin which was confirmed by the therapeutic failure of leptin in a clinical trial to treat obesity [65]. The leptin resistance of human obesity meant that the therapeutic potential of leptin as an anti-obesity agent went from a multi-million dollar enterprise in the late 1990s to an avenue with little therapeutic or financial mileage. The resurrection of leptin as an anti-obesity agent has come through work investigating the co-administration of leptin with a second agent in an attempt to overcome leptin resistance. Two such strategies appear promising in early trials. The first is the combination of leptin with amylin, a peptide that is co-secreted with insulin by pancreatic beta cells and which has been found to restore leptin responsiveness in DIO rats [66] and in addition resulted in a 12.7% mean weight loss in obese humans over the course of a 6-month trial [67]. The second approach has been to define leptin resistance as the manifestation of a state of endoplasmic reticulum (ER) stress, which activates a signalling cascade known as the unfolded protein response [68], a situation which has been implicated in the genesis of several metabolic diseases. Recent work has reported that celastrol, extracted from the roots of the *Tripterygium wilfordii*, restores leptin sensitivity in DIO mice by reducing ER stress in the hypothalamus, resulting in a reduction in food intake and body weight, an effect that is not seen in leptin-null or leptin-receptor deficient mice [69].

An altogether different approach to weight loss has followed on from the discovery that human adults possess metabolically active brown adipose tissue (BAT) [70,71]. This finding presented a new target for the treatment of obesity different to that of appetite suppression and satiety. BAT is a mitochondria-rich tissue and is a key site of adaptive thermogenesis and energy expenditure. In response to a cold stress, sympathetic stimulation of the tissue results in the increased expression and activation of uncoupling protein-1 (UCP-1) which dissipates the proton gradient across the inner mitochondrial membrane leading to the production of heat rather than ATP [72]. In general terms there are two approaches to targeting BAT to treat obesity. The first is to increase the amount of brown fat in an organism, an approach based on the observation that the amount of BAT present in adult humans is inversely correlated with BMI [73]. The second approach is based on the use of agents which enhance BAT activity as a way to increase basal energy expenditure. In addition certain stimuli, for example beta adrenergic stimulation or cold exposure can result in a browning process whereby brown in white (brite) or beige adipocytes are found within white adipose tissue deposits which could have therapeutic potential [74]. Time will tell if BAT will prove to be an efficacious target in the treatment of obesity. Historical attempts to increase energy expenditure using thyroid hormones or the uncoupler of oxidative phosphorylation 2,4-dinitrophenol (DNP), were not pursued due to toxicity. DNP continues to be used illicitly for weight loss and has resulted in deaths from hyperthermia [75].

CONCLUSION

Work to develop anti-obesity drugs remains ongoing. As our understanding of the physiological pathways that regulate food intake and energy expenditure improves, so too will our ability to develop agents that target these systems. Ultimately, there is unlikely to be a magic bullet for the treatment of obesity. Instead, the cumulative effects of targeting several different regulatory pathways, as we routinely do in the management of other chronic metabolic diseases, may in the future finally yield some of the success that has so far eluded us in the drug treatment of obesity.

Key points for clinical practice

- The obesity epidemic shows no sign of abating and the condition now affects up to 23% of adults in the WHO European region.
- To date, bariatric surgery remains the only efficacious treatment for obesity resulting in long-term weight loss associated with improvements in cardiovascular and metabolic risk.
- The principle of anti-obesity drug development is that the agent should reduce appetite, decrease the absorption of food, increase energy expenditure or some combination of all three.

- In the quest to develop safe effective anti-obesity pharmacotherapy, several drugs have been removed from the market in the wake of side effects and patient deaths.
- Drugs which are currently used for the treatment of obesity result in some weight loss but are often associated with significant side effects.
- Work to re-create the gut hormone effects of bariatric surgery without the need for the operation itself (medical bypass) has led to the development of single molecule hybrids of either two or three gut hormone receptor agonists which mimic the synergistic effects of multiple gut hormones working in concert after surgery.

REFERENCES

1.   Parliamentary Office of Science and Technology. Postnote Number 495: Obesity Treatments. London: Parliamentary Office of Science and Technology; 2015.
2.   Gortmaker SL, Must A, Perrin J, Sobol AM, Dietz WH. Social and economic consequences of overweight in adolescence and young adulthood. N Engl J Med 1993; 329:1008–1012.
3.   Staffieri JR. A study of social stereotype of body image in children. J Pers Soc Psychol 1967; 7:101–104.
4.   Latner JD, Stunkard AJ. Getting worse: the stigmatization of obese children. Obes Res 2003; 11:452–456.
5.   Counterweight Project Team. Evaluation of the counterweight programme for obesity management in primary care: a starting point for continuous improvement. Br J Gen Pract 2008; 58:548–554.
6.   Jennings A, Hughes CA, Kumaravel B, et al. Evaluation of a multidisciplinary Tier 3 weight management service for adults with morbid obesity, or obesity and comorbidities, based in primary care. Clin Obes 2014; 4:254–266.
7.   Sjostrom L, Lindroos AK, Peltonen M, et al. Lifestyle, diabetes, and cardiovascular risk factors 10 years after bariatric surgery. N Engl J Med 2004; 351:2683–2693.
8.   Bray GA. Use and abuse of appetite-suppressant drugs in the treatment of obesity. Ann Intern Med 1993; 119:707–713.
9.   Weintraub M. Long-term weight control: the National Heart, Lung, and Blood Institute funded multimodal intervention study. Clin Pharmacol Ther 1992; 51:581–585.
10. Connolly HM, Crary JL, McGoon MD, et al. Valvular heart disease associated with fenfluramine-phentermine. N Engl J Med 1997; 337:581–588.
11. Roth BL. Drugs and valvular heart disease. N Engl J Med 2007; 356:6–9.
12. SoRelle R. Diet drug maker agrees to $3.75 billion settlement. Circulation 1999; 100:e133–134.
13. Weisberg SP, Hunter D, Huber R, et al. CCR2 modulates inflammatory and metabolic effects of high-fat feeding. J Clin Invest 2006; 116:115–124.
14. Li M, Cheung BM. Pharmacotherapy for obesity. Br J Clin Pharmacol 2009; 68:804–810.
15. James WP, Caterson ID, Coutinho W, et al. Effect of sibutramine on cardiovascular outcomes in overweight and obese subjects. N Engl J Med 2010; 363:905–917.
16. Guerciolini R. Mode of action of orlistat. Int J Obes Relat Metab Disord 1997; 21:S12–23.
17. Sjostrom L, Rissanen A, Andersen T, et al. Randomised placebo-controlled trial of orlistat for weight loss and prevention of weight regain in obese patients. European Multicentre Orlistat Study Group. Lancet 1998; 352:167–172.
18. Padwal R, Li SK, Lau DC. Long-term pharmacotherapy for overweight and obesity: a systematic review and meta-analysis of randomized controlled trials. Int J Obes Relat Metab Disord 2003; 27:1437–1446.
19. Padwal R, Kezouh A, Levine M, Etminan M. Long-term persistence with orlistat and sibutramine in a population-based cohort. Int J Obes (Lond) 2007; 31:1567–1570.
20. McCarthy WJ. Orlistat and weight loss. Lancet 1998; 352:1473; author reply 1474.
21. Food and Drug Administration. Questions and Answers: Orlistat and Severe Liver Injury. New Hampshire, MA: Food and Drug Administration; 2010.
22. National Institute for Health and Care Excellence (NICE). Obesity: identification, assessment and management of overweight and obesity in children, young people and adults, 2014.
23. Eissele R, Goke R, Willemer S, et al. Glucagon-like peptide-1 cells in the gastrointestinal tract and pancreas of rat, pig and man. Eur J Clin Invest 1992; 22:283–291.

24. Herrmann C, Goke R, Richter G, et al. Glucagon-like peptide-1 and glucose-dependent insulin-releasing polypeptide plasma levels in response to nutrients. Digestion 1995; 56:117–126.

25. Drucker DJ. The biology of incretin hormones. Cell Metab 2006; 3:153–165.

26. Verdich C, Flint A, Gutzwiller JP, et al. A meta-analysis of the effect of glucagon-like peptide-1 (7-36) amide on ad libitum energy intake in humans. J Clin Endocrinol Metab 2001; 86:4382–4389.

27. Naslund E, Barkeling B, King N, et al. Energy intake and appetite are suppressed by glucagon-like peptide-1 (GLP-1) in obese men. Int J Obes Relat Metab Disord 1999; 23:304–311.

28. Dockray GJ. Enteroendocrine cell signalling via the vagus nerve. Curr Opin Pharmacol 2013; 13954–958.

29. Kanse SM, Kreymann B, Ghatei MA, Bloom SR. Identification and characterization of glucagon-like peptide-1 7-36 amide-binding sites in the rat brain and lung. FEBS Lett 1988; 241:209–212.

30. Turton MD, O'Shea D, Gunn I, et al. A role for glucagon-like peptide-1 in the central regulation of feeding. Nature 1996; 379:69–72.

31. Shughrue PJ, Lane MV, Merchenthaler I. Glucagon-like peptide-1 receptor (GLP1-R) mRNA in the rat hypothalamus. Endocrinology 1996; 137:5159–5162.

32. Hayes MR, Bradley L, Grill HJ. Endogenous hindbrain glucagon-like peptide-1 receptor activation contributes to the control of food intake by mediating gastric satiation signaling. Endocrinology 2009; 150: 2654–2659.

33. Nauck MA, Niedereichholz U, Ettler R, et al. Glucagon-like peptide 1 inhibition of gastric emptying outweighs its insulinotropic effects in healthy humans. Am J Physiol 1997; 273:E981–988.

34. Imeryuz N, Yegen BC, Bozkurt A, et al. Glucagon-like peptide-1 inhibits gastric emptying via vagal afferent-mediated central mechanisms. Am J Physiol 1997; 273:G920–927.

35. Abbott CR, Small CJ, Kennedy AR,. Blockade of the neuropeptide Y Y2 receptor with the specific antagonist BIIE0246 attenuates the effect of endogenous and exogenous peptide YY(3-36) on food intake. Brain Res 2005; 1043:139–144.

36. Astrup A, Rossner S, van Gaal L, et al. Effects of liraglutide in the treatment of obesity: a randomised, double-blind, placebo-controlled study. Lancet 2009; 374:1606-1616.

37. Amori RE, Lau J, Pittas AG. Efficacy and safety of incretin therapy in type 2 diabetes: systematic review and meta-analysis. JAMA 2007; 298:194–206.

38. Pi-Sunyer X, Astrup A, Fujioka K, et al. A randomized, controlled trial of 3.0 Mg of liraglutide in weight management. N Engl J Med 2015; 373:11–22.

39. Greenway FL, Whitehouse MJ, Guttadauria M, et al. Rational design of a combination medication for the treatment of obesity. Obesity (Silver Spring) 2009; 17:30–39.

40. Greenway FL, Dunayevich E, Tollefson G, et al. Comparison of combined bupropion and naltrexone therapy for obesity with monotherapy and placebo. J Clin Endocrinol Metab 2009a; 94:4898–4906.

41. Greenway FL, Fujioka K, Plodkowski RA, et al. Effect of naltrexone plus bupropion on weight loss in overweight and obese adults (COR-I): a multicentre, randomised, double-blind, placebo-controlled, phase 3 trial. Lancet 2010; 376:595–605.

42. Wadden TA, Foreyt JP, Foster GD, et al. Weight loss with naltrexone SR/bupropion SR combination therapy as an adjunct to behavior modification: the COR-BMOD trial. Obesity (Silver Spring) 2011; 19:110–120.

43. Apovian CM, Aronne L, Rubino D, et al. A randomized, phase 3 trial of naltrexone SR/bupropion SR on weight and obesity-related risk factors (COR-II). Obesity (Silver Spring) 2013; 21:935–943.

44. Hollander P, Gupta AK, Plodkowski R, et al. Effects of naltrexone sustained-release/bupropion sustained-release combination therapy on body weight and glycemic parameters in overweight and obese patients with type 2 diabetes. Diabetes Care 2013; 36:4022–4029.

45. Chan EW, He Y, Chui CS, et al. Efficacy and safety of lorcaserin in obese adults: a meta-analysis of 1-year randomized controlled trials (RCTs) and narrative review on short-term RCTs. Obes Rev 2013; 14:383–392.

46. Smith SR, Weissman NJ, Anderson CM, et al. Multicenter, placebo-controlled trial of lorcaserin for weight management. N Engl J Med 2010; 363:245–256.

47. European Medicines Agency. Withdrawal of the marketing authorisation application for Belviq (lorcaserin): questions and answers. London: European Medicines Agency, 2013.

48. Verrotti A, Scaparrotta A, Agostinelli S, et al. Topiramate-induced weight loss: a review. Epilepsy Res 2011; 95189–199.

49. Gadde KM, Allison DB, Ryan DH. Effects of low-dose, controlled-release, phentermine plus topiramate combination on weight and associated comorbidities in overweight and obese adults (CONQUER): a randomised, placebo-controlled, phase 3 trial. Lancet 2011; 377:1341–1352.

50. Allison DB, Gadde KM, Garvey WT, et al. Controlled-release phentermine/topiramate in severely obese adults: a randomized controlled trial (EQUIP). Obesity (Silver Spring) 2012; 20;330–342.

51. Garvey WT, Ryan DH, Look M, et al. Two-year sustained weight loss and metabolic benefits with controlled-release phentermine/topiramate in obese and overweight adults (SEQUEL): a randomized, placebo-controlled, phase 3 extension study. Am J Clin Nutr 2012; 95:297–308.

52. European Medicines Agency. Refusal of the marketing authorsation for Qsiva (phentermine/topiramate): outcome of re-examination. London: European Medicines Agency; 2013.

53. Wolfe SM. When EMA and FDA decisions conflict: differences in patients or in regulation? Br Med J 2013; 347:f5140.

54. Woloshin S, Schwartz LM. The new weight-loss drugs, lorcaserin and phentermine-topiramate: slim pickings? JAMA Intern Med 174: 615–619.

55. Smith SR. Drug treatment of obesity. JAMA Intern Med 2014; 174:1414–1415.

56. Kyle TK, Nadglowski J Jr. Drug treatment of obesity. JAMA Intern Med 2014; 174:1414.

57. Day JW, Ottaway N, Patterson JT, et al. A new glucagon and GLP-1 co-agonist eliminates obesity in rodents. Nat Chem Biol 2009; 5:749–757.

58. Finan B, Ma T, Ottaway N, Muller TD, et al. Unimolecular dual incretins maximize metabolic benefits in rodents, monkeys, and humans. Sci Transl Med 2013; 5:209ra151.

59. Finan B, Yang B, Ottaway N, et al. A rationally designed monomeric peptide triagonist corrects obesity and diabetes in rodents. Nat Med 2015; 21:27–36.

60. Zhang Y, Proenca R, Maffei M, et al. Positional cloning of the mouse obese gene and its human homologue. Nature 1994; 372:425–432.

61. Pelleymounter MA, Cullen MJ, Baker MB, et al. Effects of the obese gene product on body weight regulation in ob/ob mice. Science 1995; 269:540–543.

62. Maffei M, Halaas J, Ravussin E, et al. Leptin levels in human and rodent: measurement of plasma leptin and ob RNA in obese and weight-reduced subjects. Nat Med 1995; 1:1155–1161.

63. Frederich RC, Hamann A, Anderson S, et al. Leptin levels reflect body lipid content in mice: evidence for diet-induced resistance to leptin action. Nat Med 1995; 1:1311–1314.

64. Considine RV, Sinha MK, Heiman ML, et al. Serum immunoreactive-leptin concentrations in normal-weight and obese humans. N Engl J Med 1996; 334:292–295.

65. Heymsfield SB, Greenberg AS, Fujioka K, et al. Recombinant leptin for weight loss in obese and lean adults: a randomized, controlled, dose-escalation trial. JAMA 1999; 282:1568–1575.

66. Roth JD, Roland BL, Cole RL, et al. Leptin responsiveness restored by amylin agonism in diet-induced obesity: evidence from nonclinical and clinical studies. Proc Natl Acad Sci USA 2008; 105:7257–7262.

67. Ravussin E, Smith SR, Mitchell JA, et al. Enhanced weight loss with pramlintide/metreleptin: an integrated neurohormonal approach to obesity pharmacotherapy. Obesity (Silver Spring) 2009; 17:1736–1743.

68. Ron D, Walter P. Signal integration in the endoplasmic reticulum unfolded protein response. Nat Rev Mol Cell Biol 2007; 8:519–529.

69. Liu J, Lee J, Salazar Hernandez MA, Mazitschek R, Ozcan U. Treatment of obesity with celastrol. Cell 2015; 161:999–1011.

70. Nedergaard J, Bengtsson T, Cannon B. Unexpected evidence for active brown adipose tissue in adult humans. Am J Physiol Endocrinol Metab 2007; 293:E444–452.

71. Virtanen KA, Lidell ME, Orava J, et al. Functional brown adipose tissue in healthy adults. N Engl J Med 2009; 360:1518–1525.

72. Lowell BB, Flier JS. Brown adipose tissue, beta 3-adrenergic receptors and obesity. Annu Rev Med 1997; 48:307-316.

73. Cypess AM, Lehman S, Williams G, et al. Identification and importance of brown adipose tissue in adult humans. N Engl J Med 2009; 360:1509–1517.

74. Wu J, Bostrom P, Sparks LM, et al. Beige adipocytes are a distinct type of thermogenic fat cell in mouse and human. Cell 2012; 150:366–376.

75. Bartlett J, Brunner M, Gough K. Deliberate poisoning with dinitrophenol (DNP): an unlicensed weight loss pill. Emerg Med J 2010; 27:159–160.

Chapter 10

Novel treatment options for diabetes mellitus

Neil E Hill, Sarah N Ali, Nick S Oliver

INTRODUCTION

The array of medications, technology and interventions to assist improving glycaemic control in people with diabetes has grown considerably in the recent past. From analogue insulins, which have adapted human insulin to produce favourable pharmacokinetic profiles, through to sodium-glucose transporter-2 (SGLT2) inhibitors, which block renal reabsorption of glucose, there is an ever-growing list of tools. In this chapter, we will examine the theory and evidence for these novel treatments and place them in context for practicing clinicians.

Before proceeding though, perhaps it would be wise to highlight an underlying tension. The evidence that supports the dogma of tight glycaemic control to prevent macro- and microvascular complications has been challenged by the results of several large well-conducted randomised trials. Although the Diabetes Control and Complications Trial for type 1 diabetes (DCCT) and the UK Prospective Diabetes Study for type 2 diabetes (UKPDS) unequivocally demonstrated micro- and macrovascular benefits of tight glycaemic control in people with newly diagnosed diabetes, later studies, namely ADVANCE, ACCORD and VADT, have not corroborated these early findings [1–5]. It appears that in certain groups of people with diabetes, in particular those with type 2 of more than 10 years duration, tight glycaemic control may not always be the most important factor. Instead, it could be argued that avoidance of hypoglycaemia, attention to blood pressure and cholesterol management and not smoking should take primacy. This is reflected in national guidelines, in which individualised treatment goals and glycaemic targets are recommended [6,7].

Furthermore, since the withdrawal of rosiglitazone in 2007, there has been a degree of uncertainty about the long-term safety profiles and lack of clinically important outcome data of newer agents [8,9]. For example, concerns have surfaced about the risk of pancreatitis and pancreatic cancer with GLP-1 agonists [10,11]. This underlying worry is hard to show 'evidence' for but can be seen in blogs and on internet forums where diabetologists congregate. Many, it would seem, are happier with the 'proven' agents: metformin, sulfonylureas and insulin, but even here there are difficulties in data

Neil E Hill MRCP PhD, Imperial College Healthcare NHS Trust, London, UK. Email n.hill@imperial.ac.uk (for correspondence).

Sarah N Ali MRCP, Imperial College Healthcare NHS Trust, London, UK.

Nick S Oliver FRCP, Imperial College London, London, UK.

interpretation. The cohort of people with type 2 diabetes studied in the UKDPS were (generally) older, leaner and contained a greater proportion of smokers and Caucasians than many clinicians now see in their daily practice, and the study is more than 20-years-old [2]. Similarly, the DCCT used neutral protamine hagedorn (NPH) and human insulins which are infrequently utilised now for type 1 diabetes [1]. Extrapolating results from these studies may not always be appropriate, although most would argue that until further evidence supersedes it, this is the best we have.

Put simply, it seems that evidence supports 'tight' glycaemic control for the avoidance of diabetes-related complications but we do not know how tight or in whom; and of the medications and treatments available it is not clear which of these will translate into long-term gains that matter to individuals – avoidance of heart disease, renal failure, peripheral neuropathy and loss of eyesight with an acceptable side-effect profile both in the short and longer terms. In spite of this uncertainty, the fact that we have many agents to assist our patients should be seen as a positive, whilst recognising that they must be used judiciously with appropriate explanations of the uncertainties we face.

SODIUM-GLUCOSE TRANSPORTER-2 INHIBITORS

Sodium-glucose transporter-2 inhibitors are a recently introduced class of drugs licensed for the treatment of diabetes. Glucose is freely filtered at the glomerulus and fully reabsorbed by SGLT2 at the proximal convoluted tubule (and to a lesser extent by SGLT1 in the distal tubule) until their maximum capacity is exceeded, after which some glucose will be lost in the urine. SGLT2 inhibitors act within the kidney, effectively lowering the renal glucose reabsorptive threshold, resulting in less of the filtered glucose load being reabsorbed into the blood stream and enhancing glycosuria. Interestingly endogenous glucose production is increased following SGLT2 administration (albeit to a lesser extent than urinary glucose loss, and in spite of) perhaps due to changes in glucagon-insulin ratio, although fasting glucose levels are consistently reduced [12]. Furthermore, there is some evidence that SGLT2 inhibitors shift metabolic substrate utilisation from carbohydrate towards lipid oxidation. They are therefore attractive as they have potential to limit post-prandial hyperglycaemia and promote weight loss through glycosuria, without increasing the risk of hypoglycaemia (being independent of insulin action).

The first SGLT2 inhibitor to gain regulatory approval for use in Europe was dapagliflozin in 2012, later approved by the National Institute of Clinical Excellence in June 2013 as an add-on to metformin for patients with type 2 diabetes unable to take a sulphonylurea, or in those taking insulin [13]. Dapagliflozin is available in a 10 mg dose. Since then, canagliflozin (in 100 mg and 300 mg doses) and empagliflozin (available at 10 mg and 25 mg) have been licensed and approved by NICE for use in type 2 diabetes as (i) a second agent in those taking metformin unable to have sulphonylureas, (ii) a third agent in those on metformin and a sulphonylurea or pioglitazone or (iii) in those on insulin [13].

The hypothetical benefits of SGLT2 inhibitors seem to be borne out in the evidence published to date. Indeed several recent meta-analyses and network meta-analyses have been undertaken [14–17]. These differ from one another in methodology, inclusion criteria, corrections for bias, and whether SGLT2 inhibitors were being investigated collectively or as individual drugs (of which dapagliflozin has most publications). All of the studies included in these meta-analyses were of short duration (most lasting between 12–48 weeks) and almost all were industry sponsored and therefore at high risk of bias.

adults with type 2 diabetes in combination with oral glucose-lowering drugs when these alone or combined with basal insulin provide inadequate glycaemic control. A phase III DUAL I trial compared IDegLira ($n = 834$) with degludec ($n = 414$) and liraglutide ($n = 415$) in insulin-naïve patients with type 2 diabetes, showing a reduction in HbA1c 1.9% with IDegLira, contrasted with 1.4% for degludec and 1.3% with liraglutide. Fewer patients on IDegLira reported nausea compared to liraglutide alone. The number of hypoglycaemic episodes per patient year was 1.8 for IDegLira, 0.2 for liraglutide, and 2.6 for degludec, with similar rates of severe hypoglycaemia between all groups [38]. Likewise, a phase II DUAL II trial with IDegLira achieved superior glycaemic control compared to degludec (−1.9% versus −0.9%, $p <0.0001$) and significant weight loss ($p <0.0001$). Hypoglycaemic incidence was comparable between the two groups but nausea was higher in those treated with IDegLira [39].

ULTRA-FAST ACTING INSULIN AND CO-USE OF RHUPH20 HYALURONIDASE

Endogenous insulin response to a meal is very fast and current rapid-acting analogues are unable to achieve the same profile. Recombinant human hyaluronidase (rHuPH20) has been developed to increase the absorption and dispersion of rapid-acting insulin analogues. Its action is against hyaluronan found in subcutaneous tissues, which normally impedes the absorption of injected insulin. Thus by transiently improving the absorption of injected insulin, results a faster, shorter time–action profile closely mimicking normal physiology [40–42]. Studies with rHuPH20 show improved postprandial glucose control in test meal settings and it is well-tolerated with no adverse events reported. However, long-term safety data are lacking [43].

SENSOR-AUGMENTED PUMP THERAPY

Sensor-augmented pump therapy is the simultaneous use of real-time continuous glucose monitoring with an insulin pump, usually with the continuous glucose sensor data wirelessly transmitted to the pump display.

In basic sensor-augmented pump systems, glucose sensor data are not utilised by the pump to adapt insulin delivery, even during hypo- or hyperglycaemia. In the first treat-to-target study of sensor-augmented pump hypoglycaemia, area-under-the-curve was reduced with sensor use while HbA1c was unchanged [44]. As with subsequent studies, and in keeping with the real-time CGM data, benefit was associated with sensor usage [45,46]. The RealTrend study assessed the impact of adding CGM to insulin pump therapy at initiation and, again, found an HbA1c benefit at 6 months for those that used the CGM for $\geq 70\%$ of the time (HbA1c −0.96% versus −0.55%, $p < 0.004$) [47].

The STAR3 study demonstrated a significant reduction in HbA1c over 12 months with sensor-augmented pump compared with multiple dose injection regimens (HbA1c −0.8% versus −0.2%, $p < 0.001$), but the absence of a group using insulin pump therapy with self-monitoring of blood glucose alone makes the study difficult to interpret and of limited use [48]. A later analysis of which participants benefitted most from sensor-augmented pump therapy in STAR3 showed it was those with a higher HbA1c, those who were older and those diagnosed at an older age [49]. The use of sensor-augmented pump therapy also had a positive effect on hypoglycaemia fear and treatment satisfaction for people with type 1 diabetes and their caregivers [50].

In more advanced systems, the insulin infusion is stopped in response to hypoglycaemia or in advance of impending hypoglycaemia predicted by the glucose falling. The insulin infusion is suspended for either a fixed time (of up to 2 hours) or until the glucose rises above a threshold. Initial 'low glucose suspend' systems suspended insulin delivery for 2 hours at a hypoglycaemic threshold.

This reduced exposure to hypoglycaemia in an early study [51]. A subsequent exercise study in the clinical research facility showed a significant reduction in the duration and severity of hypoglycaemia when using low glucose suspend, without a late rebound hyperglycaemic excursion [52]. A randomised controlled study of a low glucose suspend sensor augmented pump system over 3 months has shown a reduction in nocturnal hypoglycaemia without an adverse impact on HbA1c and real-world data confirm this and reinforce the dose-dependent nature of the benefits gained from using continuous glucose sensors [53,54].

Newer systems include a predictive algorithm, enabling suspension of the insulin infusion in advance of hypoglycaemia and further data illustrating the impact on hypo- and hyperglycaemia are expected.

CONCLUSION

In summary, there have been a large number of novel treatment options released and approved in the recent past, and more are being developed. SGLT2 inhibitors are licensed for type 2 diabetes and impair renal tubular reabsorption of glucose, causing glycosuria with moderate improvements in HbA1c, and lowering of blood pressure. There are concerns about the risk of euglycaemic DKA in people with low insulin secretion or type 1 diabetes. However, the reduced cardiovascular and overall mortality seen with empagliflozin in one large multi-center study [22], if replicated makes interesting reading for physicians all too familiar with drug withdrawals and serious adverse side effects seen in other diabetes medications released to great fanfare. Insulins delivered via novel routes such as inhaled or buccal, currently still undergoing trials and may hold some promise, especially for people with needle phobias. Very long-acting insulins are already available, and provide greater flexibility in the timings of basal insulin administration and potentially lower nocturnal hypoglycaemia. Sensor-augmented insulin pump therapy for people with type 1 diabetes has been shown to improve HbA1c and reduce nocturnal hypoglycaemia.

Key points for clinical practice

- There is an increasing number of novel treatment options for diabetes.
- SGLT2 inhibitors have been shown to improve mortality but have been associated with a number of cases of euglycaemic DKA.
- Very long-acting, ultra-fast acting, buccal and inhaled insulins are being tested or have recently been released but currently lack long-term data.
- Sensor augmented insulin pump therapy can improve HbA1c and reduce nocturnal hypoglycaemia.

REFERENCES

1. The Diabetes Control and Complications Trial Research Group. The effect of intensive treatment of diabetes on the development and progression of long-term complications in insulin-dependent diabetes mellitus. N Engl J Med 1993; 329:977–986.
2. UK Prospective Diabetes Study (UKPDS) Group. Effect of intensive blood-glucose control with metformin on complications in overweight patients with type 2 diabetes (UKPDS 34). Lancet 1998; 352:854–865.
3. ADVANCE Collaborative Group. Intensive blood glucose control and vascular outcomes in patients with type 2 diabetes. N Engl J Med 2008; 358:2560–2572.
4. Action to Control Cardiovascular Risk in Diabetes Study Group. Effects of intensive glucose lowering in type 2 diabetes. N Engl J Med 2008; 358:2545–2559.
5. Duckworth W, Abraira C, Moritz T, et al Glucose control and vascular complications in veterans with type 2 diabetes. N Engl J Med 2009; 360:129–139.
6. National Institute of Clinical Excellence. Type 2 diabetes in adults: management. NICE guidelines [NG28]. Manchester: National Institute of Clinical Excellence, 2015.
7. American Diabetes Association. Standards of medical care in diabetes – 2015. Diabetes Care. 2015; 38:S33–S40.
8. Nissen SE, Wolski K. Effect of rosiglitazone on the risk of myocardial infarction and death from cardiovascular causes. N Engl J Med 2007; 356:2457–2471.
9. US Food and Drug Administration. FDA Issues Safety Alert on Avandia. Maryland, USA: US Food and Drug Administration, 2007.
10. Butler AE, Campbell-Thompson M, Gurlo T, et al. Marked expansion of exocrine and endocrine pancreas with incretin therapy in humans with increased exocrine pancreas dysplasia and the potential for glucagon-producing neuroendocrine tumors. Diabetes 2013; 62:2595–2604.
11. Egan AG, Blind E, Dunder K, et al. Pancreatic safety of incretin-based drugs – FDA and EMA assessment. N Engl J Med 2014; 370:794–797.
12. Cefalu T. Paradoxical insights into whole body metabolic adaptations following SGLT2 inhibition. JCI. 2014; 124:485–487.
13. National Institute for Health and Clinical Excellence. Dapagliflozin in combination therapy for treating type 2 diabetes. London: National Institute for Health and Clinical Excellence, 2013.
14. Zhang M, Zhang L, Wu B, et al. Dapagliflozin treatment for type 2 diabetes: a systematic review and meta-analysis of randomized controlled trials. Diabetes Metab Res Rev 2014; 30:204–2021.
15. Vasilakou D, Karagiannis T, Athanasiadou E, et al. Sodium-glucose cotransporter 2 inhibitors for type 2 diabetes: a systematic review and meta-analysis. Ann Intern Med 2013; 159:262–274.
16. Sun YN, Zhou Y, Chen X, et al. The efficacy of dapagliflozin combined with hypoglycaemic drugs in treating type 2 diabetes mellitus: meta-analysis of randomised controlled trials. BMJ Open 2014; 4:e004619.
17. Yang XP, Lai D, Zhong XY, et al. Efficacy and safety of canagliflozin in subjects with type 2 diabetes: systematic review and meta-analysis. Eur J Clin Pharmacol 2014; 70:1149–1158.
18. Gilbert RE. The perils of clinical trials. Kidney Int 2014; 85:745–747.
19. Liakos A, Karagiannis T, Bekiari E, et al. Update on long-term efficacy and safety of dapagliflozin in patients with type 2 diabetes mellitus. Ther Adv Endocrinol Metab 2015; 6:61–67.
20. Peters AL, Buschur EO, Buse JB, et al. Euglycemic Diabetic Ketoacidosis: A Potential Complication of Treatment With Sodium-Glucose Cotransporter 2 Inhibition. Diabetes Care 2015; 38:1687–1693.
21. Henry RR, Rosenstock J, Edelman S, et al. Exploring the potential of the SGLT2 inhibitor dapagliflozin in type 1 diabetes: a randomized, double-blind, placebo-controlled pilot study. Diabetes Care 2015; 38:412–419.
22. Zinman B, Wanner C, Lachin JM, et al. Empagliflozin, Cardiovascular Outcomes, and Mortality in Type 2 Diabetes. N Engl J Med 2015; 373:2117–2128.
23. Holden SE, Gale EA, Jenkins-Jones S, et al. How many people inject insulin? UK estimates from 1991 to 2010. Diabetes Obes Metab 2014; 16:553–559.
24. Karter AJ, Subramanian U, Saha C, et al. Barriers to insulin initiation. The translating research into action for diabetes insulins starts projects. Diabetes Care 2010; 33:733–735.

25. Majumdar SR, Hemmelgarn BR, Lin M, et al. Hypoglycaemia associated with hospitalisation and adverse events in older people. Population-based cohort study. Diabetes Care 2013; 36:3585–590.
26. Rosenstock J, Lorber DL, Gnudi L, et al. Prandial inhaled insulin plus basal insulin glargine versus twice daily biaspart insulin for type 2 diabetes: a multicentre randomised trial. Lancet 2010; 375:2244–553.
27. Seewoodhary J, Phooi Yew Wong S. New Insulins for diabetes. Practical Diabetes 2015; 32:93–98.
28. Pittas AG, Westcott GP, Balk EM. Efficacy, safety, and patient acceptability of Technosphere inhaled insulin for people with diabetes: a systematic review and meta-analysis. Lancet Diabetes Endocrinol 2015; 3:886–894.
29. Kapsner P, Bergenstal RM, Rendell M, et al. Comparative efficacy and safety of Technosphere insulin and a rapid acting analogue both given with glargine in subjects with type 1 diabetes mellitus in a 52-week study. Diabetologia 2009; 52:S386.
30. Raz I, Dubinsky A, Kidron M, et al. Addition of Oralin at meal-timmes in subjects with type 2 diabetes maintained on glargine + metformin – a comparison with placebo. American Diabetes Association annual meeting 2005 (abstract number 2063-P0).
31. Guevara-Aguiree J, Guevara-Aguirre M, Saavedra J, et al. Comparison of pre-prandial s.c. regular insulin vs prandial oral insulin in adult type 1 DM subjects receiving basal S.C. twice daily isophane (NPH). American Diabetes Association annual meeting 2007 (abstract number 0474-P).
32. Bergenstal RM, Blevins TC, Morrow LA, et al. A randomised controlled study of once daily LY2605541, a novel long-acting basal insulin vs. insulin glargine in basal insulin treated patients with type 2 diabetes. Diabetes care 2012; 35:2140–2147.
33. Rosenstock J, Bergenstal RM, Blevins TC, et al. Better glycemic control and weight loss with the novel long-acting basal insulin LY2605541 compared with insulin glargine in type 1 diabetes: a randomized, crossover study. Diabetes Care 2013; 36:522–528.
34. Tresiba. Committee for Medicinal Products for Human Use (CHMP) assessment report. European Medicines Agency, 2012.
35. Rodbard HW, Gough S, Lane W, et al. Reduced risk of hypoglycemia with insulin degludec versus insulin glargine in patients with type 2 diabetes requiring high doses of basal insulin: a meta-analysis of 5 randomized begin trials. Endocr Pract 2014; 20:285–292.
36. Rodbard HW, Cariou B, Zinman B, et al. Comparison of insulin degludec with insulin glargine in insulin-naive subjects with Type 2 diabetes: a 2-year randomized, treat-to-target trial. Diabet Med 2013; 30:1298–1304.
37. Bode BW, Buse JB, Fisher M, et al. Insulin degludec improves glycaemic control with lower nocturnal hypoglycaemia risk than insulin glargine in basal-bolus treatment with mealtime insulin aspart in Type 1 diabetes (BEGIN((R)) Basal-Bolus Type 1): 2-year results of a randomized clinical trial. Diabet Med 2013; 30:1293–1297.
38. Gough SC, Bode B, Woo V, et al. JB; NN9068-3697 (DUAL-I) trial investigators. Efficacy and safety of a fixed-ratio combination of insulin degludec and liraglutide (IDegLira) compared with its components given alone: results of a phase 3, open-label, randomised, 26-week, treat-to-target trial in insulin-naive patients with type 2 diabetes. Lancet Diabetes Endocrinol 2014; 2:885–893.
39. Buse JB, Vilsbøll T, Thurman J, et al Contribution of liraglutide in the fixed ratio combination of insulin degludec and liraglutdie (IDegLira). Diabetes Care 2014; 37:2926–2933.
40. Frost GI. Recombinant human hyaluronidase (rHuPH20): an enabling platform for subcutaneous drug and fluid administration. Expert Opin Drug Deliv 2007; 4:427–440.
41. Vaughn DE, Yocum RC, Muchmore DB, et al. Accelerated pharmacokinetics and glucodynamics of prandial insulins injected with recombinant human hyaluronidase. Diabetes Technol Ther 2009; 11:345–352.
42. Vaughn DE, Muchmore DB. Use of recombinant human hyaluronidase to accelerate rapid insulin analogue absorption: experience with subcutaneous injection and continuous infusion. Endocr Pract 2011; 17:914–921.
43. Hompesch M, Muchmore DB, Morrow L, et al. Accelerated insulin pharmacokinetics and improved postprandial glycemic control in patients with type 1 diabetes after coadministration of prandial insulins with hyaluronidase. Diabetes Care 2011; 34:666–668.
44. Hirsch IB, Abelseth J, Bode BW, et al. Sensor-augmented insulin pump therapy: results of the first randomized treat-to-target study. Diabetes Technol Ther 2008; 10:377–383.
45. O'Connell M, Donath S, O'Neal DN, et al. Glycaemic impact of patient-led use of sensor-guided pump therapy in type 1 diabetes: a randomised controlled trial. Diabetologia 2009; 52:1250–1257.

46. Juvenile Diabetes Research Foundation Continuous Glucose Monitoring Study Group, Tamborlane WV, Beck RW, Bode BW, et al. Continuous glucose monitoring and intensive treatment of type 1 diabetes. N Engl J Med 2008; 359:1464–1476.

47. Raccah D, Sulmont V, Reznik Y, et al. Incremental value of continuous glucose monitoring when starting pump therapy in patients with poorly controlled type 1 diabetes: the RealTrend study. Diabetes Care 2009; 32:2245–2250.

48. Bergenstal RM, Tamborlane WV, Ahmann A, et al. Effectiveness of sensor-augmented insulin-pump therapy in type 1 diabetes. N Engl J Med 2010; 363:311–320.

49. Buse JB, Dailey G, Ahmann AA, et al. Baseline predictors of A1C reduction in adults using sensor-augmented pump therapy or multiple daily injection therapy: the STAR 3 experience. Diabetes Technol Ther 2011; 13:601–606.

50. Rubin RR, Peyrot M. Health-related quality of life and treatment satisfaction in the Sensor-Augmented Pump Therapy for A1C Reduction 3 (STAR 3) trial. Diabetes Technol Ther 2012; 14:143–151.

51. Danne T, Kordonouri O, Holder M, et al. Prevention of hypoglycemia by using low glucose suspend function in sensor-augmented pump therapy. Diabetes Technol Ther 2011; 13:1129–1134.

52. Garg S,Brazg RL, Bailey TS, et al. Reduction in duration of hypoglycemia by automatic suspension of insulin delivery: the in-clinic ASPIRE study. Diabetes Technol Ther 2012; 14:205–209.

53. Bergenstal RM, Klonoff DC, Garg SK, et al. ASPIRE In-Home Study Group. Threshold-based insulin-pump interruption for reduction of hypoglycemia. N Engl J Med 2013; 369:224–232.

54. Agrawal P, Zhong A, Welsh JB, et al. Retrospective Analysis of the Real-World Use of the Threshold Suspend Feature of Sensor-Augmented Insulin Pumps. Diabetes Technol Ther 2015; 17:316–319.

3